Critical Government Documents on Health Care

CRITICAL DOCUMENTS SERIES

Critical Government Documents on Health Care

DON PHILPOTT

CRITICAL DOCUMENTS SERIES

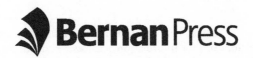

Lanham • Boulder • New York • London

RA
395
.A3
P48X
2015

Published by Bernan Press
An imprint of The Rowman & Littlefield Publishing Group, Inc.
4501 Forbes Boulevard, Suite 200, Lanham, Maryland 20706
www.rowman.com
800-865-3457; info@bernan.com

Unit A, Whitacre Mews, 26-34 Stannary Street, London SE11 4AB

Library of Congress Control Number: 2015955302

ISBN: 978-1-59888-743-3
E-ISBN: 978-1-59888-744-0

∞™ The paper used in this publication meets the minimum requirements of American National Standard for Information Sciences—Permanence of Paper for Printed Library Materials, ANSI/NISO Z39.48-1992.

Printed in the United States of America

Contents

HEART DISEASE, HEART FAILURE, AND STROKE   87

RESPIRATORY DISEASES 197

AN AGING POPULATION 207

ALZHEIMER'S AND DEMENTIA 223

Introduction

Americans are, by and large, healthier than ever before. Life expectancy for both men and women has increased over the past 25 years, although lifestyle and living longer do present health care professionals with major challenges. Rates of obesity, heart disease (high blood pressure, controlled high cholesterol), dementia, and diabetes are areas of major concern.

Average life expectancy in the United States is now 79.68 years (77.32 years for men and 81.97 years for women), based on 2015 estimates, which is up from 75.2 years in 1990. However, of 17 high-income countries studied by the National Institutes of Health in 2013, the United States had the highest or near-highest prevalence of obesity, car accidents, infant mortality, heart and lung disease, sexually transmitted infections, adolescent pregnancies, injuries, homicides, and disabilities.

Together, such issues place the United States at the bottom of the list for life expectancy. On average, a U.S. male can be expected to live almost four fewer years than those in the top-ranked country, although Americans who reach age 75 tend to live longer than those who reach that age in other developed nations.

A study by the National Research Council concluded that more than half the men who die before age 50 die from murder (19%), traffic accidents (18%), and other accidents (16%). The top causes of death for women who die before age 50 are different: 53% die from disease, and 38% die from accidents, homicide, and suicide.

The World Health Organization (WHO) reports that total health care spending in the United States was 17.9% of total Gross Domestic Product (GDP) in 2011, the highest in the world, and the Health and Human Services

Department expects that the health share of GDP will continue its historical upward trend, reaching 19.5% of GDP by 2017. Between 2000 and 2011, U.S. health care expenditures nearly doubled, growing from $1.2 trillion to $2.3 trillion, according to the Centers for Disease Control.

More Americans now have health insurance than ever before thanks to the Affordable Care Act, but millions are still uninsured and many of these go without or delay getting needed medical treatment.

The Department of Health and Human Services (HHS) uses a composite health measure that estimates not only the average length of life, but also the number of years of life people are expected to be "in good or better health, as well as free of activity limitations." Between 1997 and 2010, the number of expected high quality life years increased from 61.1 to 63.2 years for newborns.

The Department of Health and Human Services (HHS) is the United States government's principal agency for protecting the health of all Americans and providing essential human services, especially for those who are least able to help themselves. HHS is responsible for almost a quarter of all federal outlays, and it administers more grant dollars than all other federal agencies combined [CITE].

According to the HHS website, "The mission of the Department of Health and Human Services is to help provide the building blocks that Americans need to live healthy, successful lives.   We fulfill that mission every day by providing millions of children, families, and seniors with access to high-quality health care, by helping people find jobs and parents find affordable child care, by keeping the food on Americans' shelves safe and infectious diseases at bay, and by pushing the boundaries of how we diagnose and treat disease."

HHS is headed by the Secretary, who is the chief managing officer for a family of agencies, including 11 operating divisions, 10 regional offices, as well as the Office of the Secretary. Its principal divisions are:

Administration for Children and Families (ACF)

The Administration for Children and Families promotes the economic and social well-being of families, children, individuals, and communities through a range of educational and supportive programs in partnership with states, tribes, and community organizations.

Administration for Community Living (ACL)

The Administration for Community Living brings together the efforts of the Administration on Aging and the Administration on Intellectual and Developmental Disabilities to increase access to community support and resources for the unique needs of older Americans and people with disabilities across the life span.

Agency for Health Care Research and Quality (AHRQ)

The Agency for Health Care Research and Quality, as part of the Public Health Service, is responsible for supporting research designed to improve the quality of health care, reduce its costs, address patient safety and medical errors, and broaden access to essential services.

Agency for Toxic Substances and Disease Registry (ATSDR)

The Agency for Toxic Substances and Disease Registry, as part of the Public Health Service, is charged with the prevention of exposure to toxic substances and the prevention of the adverse health effects and diminished quality of life associated with exposure to hazardous substances from waste sites, unplanned releases, and other sources of pollution present in the environment.

Centers for Disease Control and Prevention (CDC)

The Centers for Disease Control and Prevention, as part of the Public Health Service, is charged with protecting the public health of the nation by providing leadership and direction in the prevention of and control of diseases and other preventable conditions and by responding to public health emergencies.

Centers for Medicare and Medicaid Services (CMS)

The Centers for Medicare and Medicaid Services combines the oversight of the Medicare program, the Federal portion of the Medicaid program and State Children's Health Insurance Program, the Health Insurance Marketplace, and related quality assurance activities.

Food and Drug Administration (FDA)

The Food and Drug Administration (FDA), as part of the Public Health Service, is charged with ensuring that food is safe, pure, and wholesome; human and animal drugs, biological products, and medical devices are safe and effective; and electronic products that emit radiation are safe.

Health Resources and Services Administration (HRSA)

The Health Resources and Services Administration (HRSA), an agency of the U.S. Department of Health and Human Services, is the primary Federal agency for improving access to health care services for people who are uninsured, isolated, or medically vulnerable.

Indian Health Service (IHS)

The Indian Health Service, as part of the Public Health Service, provides a comprehensive health services delivery system for American Indians and Alaska Natives, with opportunity for maximum tribal involvement in developing and managing programs to meet their health needs.

National Institutes of Health (NIH)

The National Institutes of Health (NIH), as part of the Public Health Service, supports biomedical and behavioral research domestically and abroad, conducts research in its own laboratories and clinics, trains promising young researchers, and promotes acquisition and distribution of medical knowledge.

Substance Abuse and Mental Health Services Administration (SAMHSA)

The Substance Abuse and Mental Health Services Administration, a part of the Public Health Service, provides national leadership to ensure that knowledge acquired is effectively used for the prevention and treatment of addictive and mental disorders. It strives to improve access and reduce barriers to high-quality, effective programs and services for individuals who suffer from or are at risk for these disorders, as well as for their families and communities.

Together these agencies are tasked with maintaining and, wherever possible, improving the nation's health.

1

The Nation's Health

In a bid to improve the nation's health HHA launched an initiative called Healthy People 2020 in December 2010. Healthy People 2020 has four goals:
- Attain high-quality, longer lives free of preventable disease, disability, injury, and premature death
- Achieve health equity, eliminate disparities, and improve the health of all groups
- Create social and physical environments that promote good health for all, and
- Promote quality of life, healthy development, and healthy behaviors across all life stages.

Healthy People 2020 tracks approximately 1,200 objectives organized into 42 topic areas, each of which represents an important public health area. These topics reflect the current status of the nation's health and wellbeing and what can be done to improve it.

The Healthy People 2020 website* describes the topics as follows:

ACCESS TO HEALTH SERVICES

Access to comprehensive, quality health care services is important for the achievement of health equity and for increasing the quality of a healthy life for everyone. The proportion of persons under age 65 who had health

---

* http://www.healthypeople.gov/2020/topicsobjectives2020/default

(medical) insurance decreased 0.6% between 2001 and 2012, from 83.6% to 83.1%, although this change was not statistically significant. Insurance coverage varied by race and ethnicity. For example, in 2012, 87.3% of the non-Hispanic white population under age 65 had health (medical) insurance, compared with 69.6% of the Hispanic or Latino population. At least 10 million formerly uninsured Americans have now gained coverage through the Affordable Health Act. However, HHS acknowledges that access to health care services in the United States is regarded as unreliable; many people do not receive the appropriate and timely care they need.

ADOLESCENT HEALTH

Adolescents (ages 10 to 19) and young adults (ages 20 to 24) make up 21 percent of the population of the United States. 8 The behavioral patterns established during these developmental periods help determine young people's current health status and their risk for developing chronic diseases in adulthood.

Although adolescence and young adulthood are generally healthy times of life, several important public health and social problems either peak or start during these years. Examples include:

- Homicide
- Suicide
- Motor vehicle crashes, including those caused by drinking and driving
- Substance use and abuse
- Smoking
- Sexually transmitted infections, including human immunodeficiency virus (HIV)
- Teen and unplanned pregnancies
- Homelessness

Because they are in developmental transition, adolescents and young adults are particularly sensitive to environmental—that is, contextual or surrounding—influences. Environmental factors, including family, peer group, school, neighborhood, policies, and societal cues, can either support or challenge young people's health and well-being. Addressing the positive development of young people facilitates their adoption of healthy behaviors and helps to ensure a healthy and productive future adult population.

The financial burdens of preventable health problems in adolescence are large and include the long-term costs of chronic diseases that are a result of behaviors begun during adolescence. For example, the annual adult health-related financial burden of cigarette smoking, which usually starts by age 18, is $193 billion.

Emerging Issues in Adolescent Health

Two important issues influence how adolescent health will be approached in the coming decade. First, the adolescent population is becoming more ethnically diverse, with rapid increases in the numbers of Hispanic and Asian American youth. The growing ethnic diversity will require cultural responsiveness to health care needs and sharpened attention to disparate health and academic outcomes, which are correlated with poverty, especially among adolescents from minority racial and ethnic groups.

The second emerging issue is the increased focus on the use of positive youth development interventions for preventing adolescent health risk behaviors. Youth development interventions can be briefly defined as the intentional process of providing all youth with the support, relationships, experiences, resources, and opportunities needed to become successful and competent adults. There is growing empirical evidence that well-designed youth development interventions can lead to positive outcomes. Ongoing, rigorous evaluation will determine what works, why it works, and how successful interventions can be applied.

ARTHRITIS, OSTEOPOROSIS, AND CHRONIC BACK CONDITIONS

Arthritis, osteoporosis, and chronic back conditions all have major effects on quality of life, the ability to work, and basic activities of daily living.

Arthritis affects 1 in 5 adults and continues to be the most common cause of disability, according to the Arthritis Foundation. It costs more than $128 billion per year and all of the human and economic costs associated with it are projected to increase over time as the population ages.

In the United States, an estimated 5.3 million people aged 50 years and older have osteoporosis. Most of these people are women, but about 0.8 million are men. Just over 34 million more people, including 12 million men, have low bone mass, which puts them at increased risk for developing osteoporosis.14 Half of all women and as many as 1 in 4 men aged 50 years and older will have an osteoporosis-related fracture in their lifetime.

About 80 percent of Americans experience low back pain (LBP) in their lifetime. It is estimated that each year:

- 15-20 percent of the population develop protracted back pain
- 2-8 percent have chronic back pain (pain that lasts more than 3 months)
- 3-4 percent of the population is temporarily disabled due to back pain
- 1 percent of the working-age population is disabled completely and permanently as a result of LBP.

Americans spend at least $50 billion each year on LBP. LBP is the:

- Second leading cause of lost work time (after the common cold)
- Third most common reason to undergo a surgical procedure
- Fifth most frequent cause of hospitalization

BLOOD DISORDERS AND BLOOD SAFETY

Blood disorders include hemoglobinopathies and abnormal bleeding and clotting. Hemoglobinopathies are inherited, lifelong blood disorders that result in abnormal hemoglobin (protein in red blood cells that carries oxygen). Complications of bleeding and clotting disorders can be prevented if the conditions are promptly recognized and treated.

Blood transfusions are lifesaving for people with severe bleeding or disorders of decreased blood production and for people undergoing surgery or recovering from severe accidents. Despite efforts by blood banks, shortages of blood product persist.

Yearly, about 1.2 million Americans develop blood clots in veins of the leg. This condition is called deep venous thrombosis (DVT). About 10 percent of people with DVT die from pulmonary embolism (PE), when a blood clot from a vein in the leg travels to the lungs, making DVT the most common preventable cause of death in hospitals. Non-symptomatic DVT is more common and can develop in nonhospitalized persons, such as long-haul air travelers.

Hemophilia is a genetic disorder that affects males and causes a deficiency (shortage) of proteins needed for normal blood clotting. For a person with hemophilia, minor injuries causing repeated joint bleeds, can lead to chronic joint disease. Chronic joint disease reduces functional capacity and causes disability. Early preventive care decreases bleeding and lessens joint disease and disability, improving quality of life.

Von Willebrand disease (vWD) is the most common blood disorder, affecting 0.6 percent to 1.3 percent of the general population. It is a bleeding disorder that affects both men and women. Women experience more symptoms because vWD increases bleeding during menstrual periods, pregnancy, and childbirth.

Hemoglobinopathies include sickle cell disease and thalassemias. These are recessive genetic disorders. This means that the disease occurs when a person inherits an abnormal gene from both parents. If both parents carry a hemoglobinopathy gene, there is a 25 percent chance that their baby will be born with the disease.

Babies born in the United States are tested at birth for common forms of hemoglobinopathies. It is estimated that at least 2 million people in the United States carry one sickle cell gene. Hemoglobinopathies are more common in people of African, Southeast Asian, and Mediterranean descent. Increased public awareness of testing for hemoglobinopathy genes (or carrier status) may increase awareness of risks for carriers and their children, and affect health-related decisions.

CANCER

Continued advances in cancer research, detection, and treatment have resulted in a decline in both incidence and death rates for all cancers. Among people who develop cancer, more than half will be alive in 5 years. Yet, cancer remains a leading cause of death in the United States, second only to heart disease. The cancer objectives for Healthy People 2020 support monitoring trends in cancer incidence, mortality, and survival to better assess the progress made toward decreasing the burden of cancer in the United States. The objectives reflect the importance of promoting evidence-based screening for cervical, colorectal, and breast cancer by measuring the use of screening tests identified in the U.S. Preventive Services Task Force (USPSTF) recommendations. The objectives for 2020 also highlight the importance of monitoring the incidence of invasive cancer (cervical and colorectal) and late-stage breast cancer, which are intermediate markers of cancer screening success.

In the coming decade, as the number of cancer survivors approaches 12 million, understanding survivors' health status and behaviors will become increasingly important. Many cancers are preventable by reducing risk factors such as:

- Use of tobacco products
- Physical inactivity and poor nutrition
- Obesity
- Ultraviolet light exposure

Other cancers can be prevented by getting vaccinated against human papillomavirus and hepatitis B virus. Screening is effective in identifying some types of cancers including:

- Breast cancer (using mammography)
- Cervical cancer (using Pap tests)
- Colorectal cancer (using fecal occult blood testing, sigmoidoscopy, or colonoscopy)

Research shows that a recommendation from a health care provider is the most important reason patients cite for having cancer screening tests.

In the past decade, overweight and obesity have emerged as new risk factors for developing certain cancers, including colorectal, breast, uterine corpus (endometrial), and kidney cancers. The impact of the current weight trends on cancer incidence will not be fully known for several decades. However, continued focus on preventing weight gain will lead to lower rates of cancer and many chronic diseases.

CHRONIC KIDNEY DISEASE (CKD)

CKD and end-stage renal disease (ESRD) are significant public health problems in the United States and a major source of suffering and poor quality of life for those afflicted. They are responsible for premature death and exact a high economic price from both the private and public sectors. They are also very costly to treat. Nearly 25 percent of the Medicare budget is used to treat people with CKD and ESRD.

Genetic determinants have a large influence on the development and progression of CKD. It is not possible to alter a person's biology and genetic determinants; however, environmental influences and individual behaviors also have a significant influence on the development and progression of CKD. As a result, some populations are disproportionately affected.

Successful behavior modification is expected to have a positive influence on the disease.

Over the past decade, several studies have shown that proteinuria (too much protein in the urine) predicts faster progression of kidney disease to ESRD. This is especially true in people with diabetes. Diabetes is the most common cause of kidney failure.

DEMENTIAS, INCLUDING ALZHEIMER'S DISEASE

Dementia is the loss of cognitive functioning—thinking, remembering, and reasoning—to such an extent that it interferes with a person's daily life. Dementia is not a disease itself, but rather a set of symptoms. Memory loss is a common symptom of dementia, although memory loss by itself does not mean a person has dementia. Alzheimer's disease is the most common cause of dementia, accounting for the majority of all diagnosed cases.

Diagnosis of dementia is key to effective treatment and care. It is important to distinguish dementia from temporary, reversible conditions that may cause loss of cognitive functioning. Temporary, reversible conditions include:

- Series of strokes
- Side effects from medication
- Chronic alcoholism
- Some tumors and infections in the brain
- Vitamin B12 deficiency
- Dehydration

Alzheimer's disease is the 6th leading cause of death among adults aged 18 years and older, according to the National Center for Health Statistics. Estimates vary, but experts suggest that up to 5.1 million Americans aged 65 years and older have Alzheimer's disease. These numbers are predicted to more than double by 2050 unless more effective ways to treat and prevent Alzheimer's disease are found.

Dementia affects an individual's health, quality of life, and ability to live independently. It can diminish a person's ability to effectively:

- Manage medications and medical conditions
- Maintain a bank account
- Drive a car or use appliances safely
- Avoid physical injury

- Maintain social relationships
- Carry out activities of daily living, such as bathing or dressing.

People living with dementia are at greater risk for general disability and experience frequent injury from falls. Older adults with dementia are 3 times more likely to have preventable hospitalizations. As their dementia worsens, people need more health services and, oftentimes, long-term care. Many individuals requiring long-term care experience major personal and financial challenges that affect their families, their caregivers, and society.

There are important steps to take to improve the identification of and care for people with dementia. These include:

- Increasing the availability of existing effective diagnostic tools.
- Decreasing the number of people with undiagnosed dementia.
- Reducing the severity of symptoms through better medical management.
- Supporting family caregivers with social, behavioral, and legal resources.
- Encouraging healthy behaviors to reduce the risk of co-occurring conditions.

Over the past decade, there has been significant scientific progress in understanding and managing dementia, with most of the research focused on Alzheimer's disease. During the next decade, it will be important that progress be made in:

- Improving the early diagnosis of Alzheimer's disease and other dementias.
- Developing interventions to delay or prevent Alzheimer's disease and other dementias.
- Finding better ways to manage dementia when other chronic conditions are present.
- Understanding the influence of lifestyle factors on a person's risk of cognitive decline and dementia.

DIABETES

Diabetes mellitus (DM) affects an estimated 23.6 million people in the United States and is the 7th leading cause of death.19
Diabetes:

- Lowers life expectancy by up to 15 years.

- Increases the risk of heart disease by 2 to 4 times.
- Is the leading cause of kidney failure, lower limb amputations, and adult-onset blindness.

In addition to these human costs, the estimated total financial cost of DM in the United States in 2007 was $174 billion, which includes the costs of medical care, disability, and premature death.

The rate of DM continues to increase both in the United States and throughout the world. Due to the steady rise in the number of persons with DM, and possibly earlier onset of type 2 DM, there is growing concern about:

- The possibility of substantial increases in diabetes-related complications
- The possibility that the increase in the number of persons with DM and the complexity of their care might overwhelm existing health care systems
- The need to take advantage of recent discoveries on the individual and societal benefits of improved diabetes management and prevention by bringing life-saving discoveries into wider practice
- The clear need to complement improved diabetes management strategies with efforts in primary prevention among those at risk for developing DM

DM occurs when the body cannot produce or respond appropriately to insulin. Insulin is a hormone that the body needs to absorb and use glucose (sugar) as fuel for the body's cells. Without a properly functioning insulin signaling system, blood glucose levels become elevated and other metabolic abnormalities occur, leading to the development of serious, disabling complications.

Many forms of diabetes exist. The 3 common types of DM are:

- Type 2 diabetes, which results from a combination of resistance to the action of insulin and insufficient insulin production.
- Type 1 diabetes, which results when the body loses its ability to produce insulin.
- Gestational diabetes, a common complication of pregnancy. Gestational diabetes can lead to perinatal complications in mother and child and substantially increases the likelihood of cesarean section. Gestational diabetes is also a risk factor for subsequent development of type 2 diabetes after pregnancy.

Effective therapy can prevent or delay diabetic complications. However, almost 25 percent of Americans with DM are undiagnosed, and another 57 million Americans have blood glucose levels that greatly increase their risk of developing DM in the next several years. Few people receive effective preventative care, which makes DM an immense and complex public health challenge.

Four "transition points" in the natural history of diabetes health care provide opportunities to reduce the health and economic burden of DM:

- Primary prevention: movement from no diabetes to diabetes
- Testing and early diagnosis: movement from unrecognized to recognized diabetes
- Access to care for all persons with diabetes: movement from no diabetes care to access to appropriate diabetes care
- Improved quality of care: movement from inadequate to adequate care

Disparities in diabetes risk:

- People from minority populations are more frequently affected by type 2 diabetes. Minority groups constitute 25 percent of all adult patients with diabetes in the United States and represent the majority of children and adolescents with type 2 diabetes.
- African Americans, Hispanic/Latino Americans, American Indians, and some Asian Americans and Native Hawaiians and other Pacific Islanders are at particularly high risk for the development of type 2 diabetes.
- Diabetes prevalence rates among American Indians are 2 to 5 times those of whites. On average, African American adults are 1.7 times as likely and Mexican Americans and Puerto Ricans are twice as likely to have the disease as non-Hispanic whites of similar age.

Barriers to progress in diabetes care include:

- Systems problems (challenges due to the design of health care systems)
- The troubling increase in the number of people with diabetes, which may result in a decrease in the attention and resources available per person to treat DM

Evidence is emerging that diabetes is associated with additional comorbidities including:

- Cognitive impairment
- Incontinence
- Fracture risk
- Cancer risk and prognosis

The importance of both diabetes and these comorbidities will continue to increase as the population ages. Therapies that have proven to reduce microvascular and macrovascular complications will need to be assessed in light of the newly identified comorbidities.

Lifestyle change has been proven effective in preventing or delaying the onset of type 2 diabetes in high-risk individuals. Based on this, new public health approaches are emerging that may deserve monitoring at the national level. For example, the Diabetes Prevention Program demonstrated that lifestyle intervention had its greatest impact in older adults and was effective in all racial and ethnic groups.

Another emerging issue is the effect on public health of new diagnostic criteria, such as introducing the use of HbA1c for diagnosis of diabetes and high risk for diabetes, and lower thresholds for gestational diabetes. These changes may impact the number of individuals with undiagnosed diabetes and facilitate the introduction of diabetes prevention at a public health level.

Several studies have suggested that process indicators such as foot exams, eye exams, and measurement of HbA1c may not be sensitive enough to capture all aspects of quality of care that ultimately result in reduced morbidity. New diabetes quality-of-care indicators are currently under development and may help determine whether appropriate, timely, evidence-based care is linked to risk factor reduction. In addition, the scientific evidence that type 2 diabetes can be prevented or delayed has stimulated new research into the best markers and approaches for identifying high-risk individuals and the most effective ways to implement prevention programs in community settings.

Finally, it may be possible to achieve additional reduction in the risk of diabetes or its complications by influencing various behavioral risk factors, such as specific dietary choices, which have not been tested in large randomized controlled trials.

DISABILITY AND HEALTH

The U.S. Census 2000 counted 49.7 million people with some type of long-lasting condition or disability. An individual can get a disabling impairment or chronic condition at any point in life. Disability is part of human life, and an impairment or condition does not define individuals, their health, or their talents and abilities.

People with disabilities play an important and valued role in every community. All people, including people with disabilities, must have the opportunity to take part in important daily activities that add to a person's growth, development, fulfillment, and community contribution. This principle is central to all objectives outlined in this topic.

The Disability and Health objectives highlight areas for improvement and opportunities for people with disabilities to:

- Be included in public health activities.
- Receive well-timed interventions and services.
- Interact with their environment without barriers.
- Participate in everyday life activities.

Compared with people without disabilities, people with disabilities are more likely to:

- Experience difficulties or delays in getting the health care they need.
- Not have had an annual dental visit.
- Not have had a mammogram in past 2 years.
- Not have had a Pap test within the past 3 years.
- Not engage in fitness activities.
- Use tobacco.
- Be overweight or obese.
- Have high blood pressure.
- Experience symptoms of psychological distress.
- Receive less social-emotional support.
- Have lower employment rates.

Public health efforts, from the individual to the national level, can affect the health and well-being of people with disabilities. These efforts must respond to known determinants of disability and health.

There are many social and physical factors that influence the health of people with disabilities. The following 3 areas for public health action have been identified, using the International Classification of Functioning, Disability, and Health (ICF) and the 3 World Health Organization (WHO) principles of action for addressing health determinants.

  I. Improve the conditions of daily life by:
- Encouraging communities to be accessible so all can live in, move through, and interact with their environment.
- Encouraging community living.
- Removing barriers in the environment using both physical universal design concepts and operational policy shifts.

2. Address the inequitable distribution of resources among people with disabilities and those without disabilities by increasing:
- Appropriate health care for people with disabilities
- Education and work opportunities
- Social participation
- Access to needed technologies and assistive supports

3. Expand the knowledge base and raise awareness about determinants of health for people with disabilities by increasing:
- The inclusion of people with disabilities in public health data collection efforts across the lifespan
- The inclusion of people with disabilities in health promotion activities
- The expansion of disability and health training opportunities for public health and health care professionals

There are several emerging issues related to disability and health, including the need to:
- Include disability and health courses.
- Assess drug and alcohol abuse and their treatment among people with disabilities.
- Include and improve strategies for emergency preparedness and response for people with disabilities.
- Include people with disabilities in all health promotion efforts.

EARLY AND MIDDLE CHILDHOOD

There is increasing recognition in policy, research, and clinical practice communities that early and middle childhood provide the physical, cognitive, and social-emotional foundation for lifelong health, learning, and well-being. Early childhood, middle childhood, and adolescence represent the 3 stages of child development. Each stage is organized around the primary tasks of development for that period.
- Early childhood (usually defined as birth to year 8) is a time of tremendous physical, cognitive, and socio-emotional development.
- Middle childhood (usually defined as ages 6 to 12) is a time when children develop skills for building healthy social relationships and learn roles that will lay ground work for a lifetime.

Evidence shows that experiences in the 1st years of life are extremely important for a child's healthy development and lifelong learning. How a child develops during this time affects future cognitive, social, emotional, and physical development, which influences school readiness and later success in life. Research on a number of adult health and medical conditions points to predisease pathways that have their beginnings in early and middle childhood.

During early childhood, the human brain grows to 90 percent of its adult size by age three. Early childhood represents the period when young children reach developmental milestones that include:

- Emotional regulation and attachment
- Language development
- Motor skills

All of these milestones can be significantly delayed when young children experience environmental stressors and other negative risk factors. These stressors and factors can affect the brain and may seriously compromise a child's physical, social-emotional, and cognitive growth and development.

More than any other developmental period, early and middle childhood sets the stage for:

- Health literacy
- Self-discipline
- The ability to make good decisions about risky situations
- Eating habits
- Conflict negotiation

Although early and middle childhood are typically healthy ages, it is during this time that children are at risk for conditions such as:

- Asthma
- Obesity
- Dental caries
- Child maltreatment
- Developmental and behavioral disorders

While typically nonfatal, these conditions affect children, their education, and the health and well-being of the adolescents and adults they will become. The keys to understanding early and middle childhood health are recognizing the important role these periods play in adult health and well-being and focusing on conditions and illnesses that can seriously limit children's abilities to learn, grow, play, and become healthy adults.

Emerging issues in early and middle childhood include implementing and evaluating multidisciplinary public health interventions that address social determinants of health by:

- Fostering knowledgeable and nurturing families, parents, and caregivers.
- Creating supportive and safe environments in schools, communities, and homes.
- Increasing access to high-quality health care.

A stronger and more robust surveillance system is needed to provide the data to understand and plan for the health and well-being of children.

EDUCATIONAL AND COMMUNITY-BASED PROGRAMS

Educational and community-based programs play a key role in:

- Preventing disease and injury.
- Improving health.
- Enhancing quality of life.

Health status and related health behaviors are determined by influences at multiple levels: personal, organizational/institutional, environmental, and policy. Because significant and dynamic interrelationships exist among these different levels of health determinants, educational and community-based programs are most likely to succeed in improving health and wellness when they address influences at all levels and in a variety of environments/settings. Over the next decade, they will continue to contribute to the improvement of health outcomes in the United States.

Education and community-based programs and strategies are designed to reach people outside of traditional health care settings. These settings may include:

- Schools
- Worksites
- Health care facilities
- Communities

Each setting provides opportunities to reach people using existing social structures. This maximizes impact and reduces the time and resources necessary for program development. People often have high levels of contact with these settings, both directly and indirectly. Programs that combine multiple—if not all four—settings can have a greater impact than programs using only one setting. While populations reached will sometimes overlap, people who are not accessible in one setting may be in another.

Using nontraditional settings can help encourage informal information sharing within communities through peer social interaction. Reaching out to people in different settings also allows for greater tailoring of health information and education. Educational and community-based programs encourage and enhance health and wellness by educating communities on topics such as:

- Chronic diseases
- Injury and violence prevention
- Mental illness/behavioral health
- Unintended pregnancy
- Oral health
- Tobacco use
- Substance abuse
- Nutrition and obesity prevention
- Physical activity

Three emerging public health issues in the area of educational and community-based programs have been identified.

Evaluating coordinated school health programs as an intervention to reduce school dropout rates. Coordinated school health programs include:

- Comprehensive school health education
- Health services
- Physical education
- Nutrition services
- Mental health and social services
- Staff wellness
- Family/community involvement
- A healthy and safe environment

Establishing an evidence base for community health and education policy interventions to determine their impact and effectiveness.

Increasing the number and skill level of community health and other auxiliary public health workers to support the achievement of healthier communities.

These issues are important to the field of public health and warrant further research, analysis, and monitoring to fully understand their effects on educational and community-based programs.

ENVIRONMENTAL HEALTH

Humans interact with the environment constantly. These interactions affect quality of life, years of healthy life lived, and health disparities. The World Health Organization (WHO) defines environment, as it relates to health, as "all the physical, chemical, and biological factors external to a person, and all the related behaviors." Environmental health consists of preventing or controlling disease, injury, and disability related to the interactions between people and their environment.

The Healthy People 2020 Environmental Health objectives focus on 6 themes, each of which highlights an element of environmental health:

Outdoor air quality

Surface and ground water quality

Toxic substances and hazardous wastes

Homes and communities

Infrastructure and surveillance

Global environmental health

Creating health-promoting environments is complex and relies on continuing research to understand more fully the effects of exposure to environmental hazards on people's health.

Maintaining a healthy environment is central to increasing quality of life and years of healthy life. Globally, nearly 25 percent of all deaths and the total disease burden can be attributed to environmental factors. Environmental factors are diverse and far reaching. They include:

- Exposure to hazardous substances in the air, water, soil, and food
- Natural and technological disasters
- Physical hazards
- Nutritional deficiencies
- The built environment

Poor environmental quality has its greatest impact on people whose health status is already at risk. Therefore, environmental health must address the societal and environmental factors that increase the likelihood of exposure and disease.

Outdoor Air Quality

Poor air quality is linked to premature death, cancer, and long-term damage to respiratory and cardiovascular systems. Progress has been made to reduce unhealthy air emissions, but, in 2008, approximately 127 million people lived in U.S. counties that exceeded national air quality standards. Decreasing air pollution is an important step in creating a healthy environment.

Surface and Ground Water

Surface and ground water quality applies to both drinking water and recreational waters. Contamination by infectious agents or chemicals can cause mild to severe illness. Protecting water sources and minimizing exposure to contaminated water sources are important parts of environmental health.

Toxic Substances and Hazardous Wastes

The health effects of toxic substances and hazardous wastes are not yet fully understood. Research to better understand how these exposures may impact health is ongoing. Meanwhile, efforts to reduce exposures continue. Reducing exposure to toxic substances and hazardous wastes is fundamental to environmental health.

Homes and Communities

People spend most of their time at home, work, or school. Some of these environments may expose people to:

- Indoor air pollution
- Inadequate heating and sanitation
- Structural problems
- Electrical and fire hazards
- Lead-based paint hazards

These hazards can impact health and safety. Maintaining healthy homes and communities is essential to environmental health.

Infrastructure and Surveillance

Prevention of exposure to environmental hazards relies on many partners, including State and local health departments. Personnel, surveillance systems, and education are important resources for investigating and responding to disease, monitoring for hazards, and educating the public. Additional methods and greater capacity to measure and respond to environmental hazards are needed.

Global Environmental Health

Water quality is an important global challenge. Diseases can be reduced by improving water quality and sanitation and increasing access to adequate water and sanitation facilities.

Environmental health is a dynamic and evolving field. While not all complex environmental issues can be predicted, some known emerging issues in the field include:

Climate Change

Climate change is projected to impact sea level, patterns of infectious disease, air quality, and the severity of natural disasters such as floods, droughts, and storms.

Disaster Preparedness

Preparedness for the environmental impact of natural disasters as well as disasters of human origin includes planning for human health needs and the impact on public infrastructure, such as water and roadways.

Nanotechnology

The potential impact of nanotechnology is significant and offers possible improvements to:

- Disease prevention, detection, and treatment
- Electronics
- Clean energy
- Manufacturing
- Environmental risk assessment

However, nanotechnology may also present unintended health risks or changes to the environment.

The Built Environment

Features of the built environment appear to impact human health-influencing behaviors, physical activity patterns, social networks, and access to resources.

Exposure to Unknown Hazards

Finally, every year, hundreds of new chemicals are introduced to the U.S. market. It is presumed that some of these chemicals may present new, unexpected challenges to human health, and, therefore, their safety should be evaluated prior to release.

These cross-cutting issues are not yet understood well enough to inform the development of systems for measuring and tracking their impact. Further exploration is warranted. The environmental health landscape will continue to evolve and may present opportunities for additional research, analysis, and monitoring.

Blood Lead Levels

The number of children with elevated blood lead levels in the U.S. is steadily decreasing. As a result, determining stable national prevalence estimates and changes in estimated prevalence over time using NHANES is increasingly difficult. Eliminating elevated blood lead levels in children remains a goal of utmost importance to public health. The sample sizes available with the currently structured NHANES are too small to produce statistically reliable estimates and preclude the ability to have a viable target for HP2020 (see Objective 8.1). Efforts must and will continue to reduce blood lead levels and to monitor the prevalence of children with elevated blood lead levels.

FAMILY PLANNING

Family planning is one of the 10 great public health achievements of the 20th century.25 The availability of family planning services allows individuals to achieve desired birth spacing and family size, and contributes to improved health outcomes for infants, children, women, and families.

Family planning services include:

- Contraceptive and broader reproductive health services, including patient education and counseling
- Breast and pelvic examinations
- Breast and cervical cancer screening
- Sexually transmitted infection (STI) and human immunodeficiency virus (HIV) prevention education, counseling, testing, and referral
- Pregnancy diagnosis and counseling

Abstinence from sexual activity is the only 100 percent effective way to avoid unintended pregnancy. For individuals who are sexually active and do not want to become pregnant or cause a pregnancy, correct and consistent contraceptive use is highly effective at preventing unintended pregnancy. The most effective methods to prevent unintended pregnancy include long-acting reversible contraceptives such as intrauterine devices (IUDs) and contraceptive implants. Condoms protect against both unintended pregnancy and STIs, and their use should be encouraged. Both men and women should be counseled about using condoms at every act of sexual intercourse, when not in a long-term, mutually monogamous sexual relationship.

For many women, a family planning clinic is the entry point into the health care system and one they consider their usual source of care. Each year, publicly funded family planning services prevent 1.94 million unintended pregnancies, including 400,000 teen pregnancies. These services are cost-effective, saving nearly $4 in Medicaid expenditures for pregnancy-related care for every $1 spent.

Unintended pregnancies are associated with many negative health and economic consequences. Unintended pregnancies include pregnancies that are reported by women as being mistimed or unwanted. Almost half of all pregnancies in the United States are unintended. The public costs of births resulting from unintended pregnancies were $11 billion in 2006. (This figure includes costs for prenatal care, labor and delivery, post-partum care, and 1 year of infant care).

For women, negative outcomes associated with unintended pregnancy can include:

- Delays in initiating prenatal care
- Reduced likelihood of breastfeeding, resulting in less healthy children
- Maternal depression
- Increased risk of physical violence during pregnancy

Births resulting from unintended pregnancies can have negative consequences including birth defects and low birth weight. Children from unintended pregnancies are more likely to experience poor mental and physical health during childhood, and have lower educational attainment and more behavioral issues in their teen years.

The negative consequences associated with unintended pregnancies are greater for teen parents and their children. Eighty-two percent of pregnancies to mothers ages 15 to 19 are unintended. One in five unintended pregnancies each year is among teens. Teen mothers:

- Are less likely to graduate from high school or attain a GED by the time they reach age 30.
- Earn an average of approximately $3,500 less per year, when compared with those who delay childbearing until their 20s.
- Receive nearly twice as much Federal aid for nearly twice as long.

Similarly, early fatherhood is associated with lower educational attainment and lower income.

The average annual cost of teen childbearing to U.S. taxpayers is estimated at $9.1 billion, or $1,430 for each teen mother per year. Moreover, children of teen parents are more likely to have lower cognitive attainment and exhibit more behavior problems. of teen mothers are more likely to be incarcerated, and daughters are more likely to become adolescent mothers.

Unintended pregnancies occur among women of all incomes, educational levels, and ages. However, there are disparities in unintended pregnancy rates. The rates of unintended pregnancy are highest among the following groups:

- Women ages 18 to 24
- Women who were cohabiting
- Women whose income is below the poverty line

- Women with less than a high school diploma
- Black or Hispanic women

Women with lower levels of education and income, uninsured women, Latina women, and non-Hispanic black women are less likely to have access to family planning services. In addition, men are less likely to have access to and to receive family planning services than women.

Barriers to people's use of family planning services include:

- Cost of services
- Limited access to publicly funded services
- Limited access to insurance coverage
- Family planning clinic locations and hours that are not convenient for clients
- Lack of awareness of family planning services among hard-to-reach populations
- No or limited transportation
- Inadequate services for men
- Lack of youth-friendly services

Many women of reproductive age can benefit from preconception care (care before pregnancy). Preconception care has been defined as a set of interventions designed to identify and reduce risks to a woman's health and improve pregnancy outcomes through prevention and management of health conditions. Preconception care can significantly reduce birth defects and disorders caused by preterm birth.

Elements of preconception care should be integrated into every primary care visit for women of reproductive age. Preconception care must not be limited to a single visit to a health care provider, but rather be a process of care designed to meet the needs of an individual. As part of comprehensive preconception care, providers should encourage patients to develop a reproductive life plan. A reproductive life plan is a set of goals and action steps based on personal values and resources about whether and when to become pregnant and have (or not have) children. Providers also must educate patients about how their reproductive life plan impacts contraceptive and medical decision-making.

Increased awareness of the importance of preconception care can be achieved through public outreach and improved collaboration between health care providers. Currently, only 30.3 percent of women report receiving pre-pregnancy health counseling. Future efforts should promote research to further define the evidence-based standards of preconception care, determine its cost-effectiveness, and improve tracking of the proportion of women obtaining these services.

FOOD SAFETY

Foodborne illnesses are a burden on public health and contribute significantly to the cost of health care. A foodborne outbreak occurs when 2 or more cases of a similar illness result from eating the same food. In 2006, the Centers for Disease Control and Prevention (CDC) received reports of a total of 1,270 foodborne disease outbreaks, which resulted in 27,634 cases of illness and 11 deaths.

A foodborne outbreak indicates that something in the food safety system needs to be improved. The food safety system includes food:

- Production
- Processing
- Packing
- Distribution/Transportation
- Storage
- Preparation

Public health scientists investigate outbreaks to control them and to learn how to prevent similar outbreaks in the future. Success is measured in part through the reduction in outbreaks of foodborne illnesses.

Foodborne illness is a preventable and underreported public health problem. It presents a major challenge to both general and at-risk populations. Each year, millions of illnesses in the United States can be attributed to contaminated foods. Children younger than age 4 have the highest incidence of laboratory-confirmed infections from:

- Campylobacter species
- Cryptosporidium species
- Salmonella species
- Shiga toxin-producing Escherichia coli O157
- Shigella species
- Yersinia species

People older than age 50 are at greater risk for hospitalizations and death from intestinal pathogens commonly transmitted through foods. 31 Safer food promises healthier and longer lives, less costly health care, and a more resilient food industry.

Many factors determine the safety of the Nation's food supply. Improper handling, preparation, and storage practices may result in cases of foodborne illness. This can happen in processing and retail establishments and in the home.

Fewer consumers grow and prepare their own food, preferring instead either to use convenience foods purchased in supermarkets that can quickly be prepared or assembled, or to eat in restaurants. This gives them less control over the foods they eat. The processing and retail food industries continue to be challenged by:

- Large employee populations that have high rates of turnover
- Non-uniform systems for training and certifying workers
- Ability to rapidly traceback/traceforward food items of interest

In addition, changes in production practices and new sources of food, such as imports, introduce new risks.

Food hazards can enter the food supply at any point from farm to table. Many foodborne hazards cannot be detected in food when it is purchased or consumed. These hazards include microbial pathogens and chemical contaminants. In addition, a food itself can cause severe adverse reactions. In the United States, food allergy is an important problem, especially among children under age 18.

GENOMICS

There are now proven health benefits from using genetic tests and family health history to guide clinical and public health interventions.

Women with certain high-risk family health history patterns for breast and ovarian cancer can benefit from receiving genetic counseling to learn about genetic testing for BRCA1/2. For women with BRCA1/2 mutations, surgery could potentially reduce the risk of breast and ovarian cancer by 85 percent or more.

All people who are newly diagnosed with colorectal cancer should receive counseling and educational materials about genetic testing. Family members could benefit from knowing whether the colorectal cancer in their family is a hereditary form called Lynch syndrome. Screening interventions could potentially reduce the risk of colorectal cancer among men and women with Lynch syndrome by 60 percent.

Genomics plays a role in 9 of the 10 leading causes of death, including:

- Heart disease
- Cancer
- Stroke
- Diabetes
- Alzheimer's disease

For people who are at increased risk for hereditary breast and ovarian, or hereditary colorectal cancer, genetic tests may reduce their risk by guiding evidence-based interventions. Genetic tests for other leading causes of death and disability are becoming available. New recommendations are expected as the scientific evidence on which tests and interventions have health benefits is strengthened.

Traditionally, public health applications of genomics have focused on rare diseases, such as those identified through newborn screening programs. Much of the future promise of genomics rests on its application to common diseases.

More than 1,700 genetic tests are currently available, including many available directly to consumers. Genetic tests have the potential to improve health in a variety of ways by informing disease:

- Diagnosis
- Prognosis
- Risk prediction
- Prevention
- Treatment, including choice of medication and dosage

On the other hand, genetic tests that are not valid or useful have the potential to cause harm by prompting inappropriate changes in medical care based on incomplete or incorrect information.

Family health history is an important risk factor for common diseases, independent from traditional risk factors. More than 50 percent of the population is at increased risk of diabetes, cancer, or heart disease because they have close relatives with 1 or more of these diseases. Family health history has the potential to improve health by finding people who are at risk for disease in the future or who are already sick but have not been diagnosed.

Although the field of genomics is rapidly producing discoveries, there are a limited number of evidence-based recommendations for genetic tests and family health history tools. The existing recommendations, after translating them into practice, have the potential for improving health. In addition, more evaluation of the potential benefits and harms from the use of genomics is needed to guide the development of new recommendations.

As genomics discoveries lead to new opportunities to improve health through the use of genetic tests and family health history tools, important challenges need to be addressed.

It is becoming increasingly difficult for evidence-based, independent review panels to evaluate quickly and thoroughly the proposed health benefits and harms of the fast-growing number of genetic tests and family health history tools.

As the number of recommended genetic tests increases, valid and reliable national data are needed to establish baseline measures and track progress toward targets. Many tests are recommended for use in small subpopulations, making it difficult for most national health information systems, such as the National Health Interview Survey (NHIS), to monitor progress. In addition, traditional administrative data sources in the health care system typically do not capture the use of genetic tests and family health history tools. For example, current procedural terminology (CPT) codes do not allow tracking of specific genetic tests in billing records.

The development of new Healthy People objectives in genomics may be hindered by the limited availability of both evidence-based practice recommendations and national data to monitor progress.

Many opportunities and challenges for realizing the promise of genomics to improve health outcomes lie ahead, including:

- Creating and evaluating scientific evidence to support valid and useful genetic tests and family health history tools.
- Developing evidence-based practice recommendations that evaluate the net health benefit of genetic tests and family health history tools.
- Conducting research on how to translate recommendations into practice.
- Facilitating the use of valid and useful genetic tests and family health history tools to guide clinical practice, policy, and national, State, and local programs to find people who are at risk for disease, make diagnoses, and provide appropriate interventions.
- Monitoring the use of genetic tests and family health history in populations, the health outcomes related to their use, and disparities in use and outcomes.
- Adding genomic information and clinical decision support tools to electronic health records.

- Incorporating health-related genomics education in primary, secondary, undergraduate, and graduate curricula.
- Assuring the privacy and confidentiality of genomic information.

Addressing these issues will require the coordinated and collaborative efforts of both the public and private sectors

GLOBAL HEALTH

The health of the U.S. population can be affected by public health threats or events across the globe. Recent examples of this include the Ebola outbreak, the SARS epidemic and the 2009 spread of novel H1N1 influenza. Improving global health can improve health in the United States and support national and global security interests by fostering political stability, diplomacy, and economic growth worldwide.

Global health plays an increasingly crucial role in global security and the security of the U.S. population. As the world and its economies become increasingly globalized, including extensive international travel and commerce, it is necessary to think about health in a global context. Rarely a week goes by without a headline about the emergence or re-emergence of an infectious disease or other health threat somewhere in the world. The 2007 World Health Report noted that, "since the 1970s, newly emerging diseases have been identified at the unprecedented rate of one or more per year." The Institute of Medicine's 2003 report Microbial Threats to Health, stressed that the United States should enhance the global capacity for responding to infectious disease threats and should take a leadership role in promoting a comprehensive, global, real-time infectious disease surveillance system.

Rapid identification and control of emerging infectious diseases helps:

- Promote health abroad.
- Prevent the international spread of disease.
- Protect the health of the U.S. population.

The large scope of potential global public health threats is recognized in the revised International Health Regulations (IHR [2005]) with its all-hazards approach to assessing serious public health threats. These regulations are designed to prevent the international spread of diseases, while minimizing interruption of world travel and trade. They encourage countries to work together to share information about known diseases and public health events of international concern.

Global health concerns are not limited to infectious diseases. Noncommunicable diseases, especially "lifestyle" conditions, are among the leading causes of disability worldwide. These conditions include:

- Diabetes and obesity
- Mental illness
- Substance abuse/use disorders, including tobacco use

Injuries

The World Health Organization (WHO) estimates that tobacco- and smoking-related deaths will increase from 5.1 million each year to 8.3 million each year by 2030 (which will be nearly 10 percent of all deaths globally). 38

In the next 10 years, road traffic injuries are expected to become the 3rd largest contributor to the global burden of disease by 2020, with 90 percent of all deaths from road traffic injuries occurring in low-income countries.39

U.S. investments in improving health in developing countries provide significant public health benefits within the United States. Many global health issues can directly or indirectly impact the health of the United States. Outbreaks of infectious diseases, foodborne illnesses, or contaminated pharmaceuticals and other products, cannot only spread from country to country, but also impact trade and travel. The United States can also learn from the experiences of other countries. Standard health measures of life expectancy and chronic disease, including depression among adults, can be compared to other Organization for Economic and Co-operation and Development (OECD) member countries. For those countries with better health outcomes than the United States, health agencies within the United States can use these comparisons to identify ways to improve the Nation's public health.

Globally, the rate of deaths from noncommunicable causes, such as heart disease, stroke, and injuries, is growing. At the same time, the number of deaths from infectious diseases, such as malaria, tuberculosis, and vaccine-preventable diseases, is decreasing. Many developing countries must now deal with a "dual burden" of disease: they must continue to prevent and control infectious diseases, while also addressing the health threats from noncommunicable diseases and environmental health risks. As social and economic conditions in developing countries change and their health systems and surveillance improve, more focus will be needed to address noncommunicable diseases, mental health, substance abuse disorders, and, especially, injuries (both intentional and unintentional). Some countries are beginning to establish programs to address these issues. For example, Kenya has implemented programs for road traffic safety and violence prevention.

Expanding international trade introduces new health risks. A complex international distribution chain has resulted in potential international outbreaks due to foodborne infections, poor quality pharmaceuticals, and contaminated consumer goods.

The world community is finding better ways to confront major health threats. WHO has proposed new guidance and promotes cooperation between developed and developing countries on emerging health issues of global importance. The IHR require countries to develop appropriate surveillance and response capacities to address these health concerns. All of these issues will require enhanced U.S. collaboration with other countries to protect and promote better health for all.

HEALTH COMMUNICATION AND HEALTH INFORMATION TECHNOLOGY

Ideas about health and behaviors are shaped by the communication, information, and technology that people interact with every day. Health communication and health information technology (IT) are central to health care, public health, and the way our society views health. These processes make up the context and the ways professionals and the public search for, understand, and use health information, significantly impacting their health decisions and actions.

There are many ways health communication and health IT can have a positive impact on health, health care, and health equity. They include:

- Supporting shared decision-making between patients and providers.
- Providing personalized self-management tools and resources.
- Building social support networks.
- Delivering accurate, accessible, and actionable health information that is targeted or tailored.
- Facilitating the meaningful use of health IT and exchange of health information among health
- Increasing health literacy skills.
- Providing new opportunities to connect with culturally diverse and hard-to-reach populations.

- Providing sound principles in the design of programs and interventions that result in healthier behaviors.
- Increasing Internet and mobile access.

Effective use of communication and technology by health care and public health professionals can bring about an age of patient- and public-centered health information and services. By strategically combining health IT tools and effective health communication processes, there is the potential to:

- Improve health care quality and safety.
- Increase the efficiency of health care and public health service delivery.
- Improve the public health information infrastructure.
- Support care in the community and at home.
- Facilitate clinical and consumer decision-making.
- Build health skills and knowledge.

All people have some ability to manage their health and the health of those they care for. However, with the increasing complexity of health information and health care settings, most people need additional information, skills, and supportive relationships to meet their health needs.

Disparities in access to health information, services, and technology can result in lower usage rates of preventive services, less knowledge of chronic disease management, higher rates of hospitalization, and poorer reported health status.

Both public and private institutions are increasingly using the Internet and other technologies to streamline the delivery of health information and services. This results in an even greater need for health professionals to develop additional skills in the understanding and use of consumer health information.

The increase in online health information and services challenges users with limited literacy skills or limited experience using the Internet. For many of these users, the Internet is stressful and overwhelming—even inaccessible. Much of this stress can be reduced through the application of evidence-based best practices in user-centered design.

In addition, despite increased access to technology, other forms of communication are essential to ensuring that everyone, including non-Web users, is able to obtain, process, and understand health information to make good health decisions. These include printed materials, media campaigns, community outreach, and interpersonal communication.

During the coming decade, the speed, scope, and scale of adoption of health IT will only increase. Social media and emerging technologies promise to blur the line between expert and peer health information. Monitoring and assessing the impact of these new media, including mobile health, on public health will be challenging.

Equally challenging will be helping health professionals and the public adapt to the changes in health care quality and efficiency due to the creative use of health communication and health IT. Continual feedback, productive interactions, and access to evidence on the effectiveness of treatments and interventions will likely transform the traditional patient-provider relationship. It will also change the way people receive, process, and evaluate health information. Capturing the scope and impact of these changes—and the role of health communication and health IT in facilitating them—will require multidisciplinary models and data systems.

Such systems will be critical to expanding the collection of data to better understand the effects of health communication and health IT on population health outcomes, health care quality, and health disparities.

HEALTH-RELATED QUALITY OF LIFE & WELL-BEING

Health-related quality of life (HRQOL) is a multi-dimensional concept that includes domains related to physical, mental, emotional, and social functioning. It goes beyond direct measures of population health, life expectancy, and causes of death, and focuses on the impact health status has on quality of life.

A related concept of HRQOL is well-being, which assesses the positive aspects of a person's life, such as positive emotions and life satisfaction. Well-being is a relative state where one maximizes his or her physical, mental, and social functioning in the context of supportive environments to live a full, satisfying, and productive life.

HSS recognizes the importance of health-related quality of life and well-being by including it as one of the initiative's 4 overarching goals, "promoting quality of life, healthy development, and health behaviors across all life stages."

The significance of quality of life and well-being as a public health concern is not new. Since 1949, the World Health Organization (WHO) has noted that health is "a state of complete physical, mental, and social well-being and not merely an absence of disease and infirmity." In 2005,

WHO recognized the importance of evaluating and improving people's quality of life in a position paper. Because people are living longer than ever before, researchers have changed the way they examine health, looking beyond causes of death and morbidity to examine the relationship of health to the quality of an individual life.

When quality of life is considered in the context of health and disease, it's commonly referred to as health-related quality of life (HRQOL). Researchers today agree that HRQOL is multidimensional and includes domains that are related to physical, mental, emotional, and social functioning and the social context in which people live.

The first overarching goal for the Healthy People 2010 decade was to increase quality and years of healthy life. Measures of life expectancy and healthy life expectancy (HLE) were used to report on this goal for several populations, which relied on self-reported data related to health, including global health status, prevalence of certain chronic diseases, and activity limitations. For Healthy People 2020, quality of life is integral to each of the 4 overarching goals.

HHS agencies have begun to prioritize the evaluation and improvement of HRQOL, for example, http://outcomes.cancer.gov/areas/assessment/. Improvements in HRQOL have become a major focus in health research, with scientists, clinicians, and policy makers recognizing the importance of individuals' self-rated experience, beyond or in addition to objective or clinical measures of health.

Promoting well-being emphasizes a person's physical, mental, and social resources and enhances protective factors and conditions that foster health. Instead of the traditional view of prevention as only avoiding or minimizing illness and risk factors, well-being also focuses on disease resistance, resilience, and self-management.

While there are several existing measures of HRQOL and well-being in use, methodological development in this area is ongoing. Over the decade, Healthy People 2020 is approaching the measurement of health-related quality of life and well-being from a multidisciplinary perspective that encompasses 3 complementary and related domains:
- Self-rated physical and mental health
- Overall well-being
- Participation in society

Although none of these domains alone can fully represent the concept of health-related quality of life or well-being, when viewed together they will provide a more complete representation to support monitoring of the health-related quality of life and well-being of the U.S. population.

Self-Rated Physical and Mental Health

HRQOL is a subjective and multidimensional concept that includes aspects of physical, mental, and social health. For Healthy People 2020, the Patient-Reported Outcomes Measurement Information System (PROMIS) Global Health Items were identified as reliable and valid measures of self-reported physical and mental health and are currently being considered to monitor these 2 domains across the decade. PROMIS is an NIH Roadmap initiative designed to develop an electronic system to collect self-reported HRQOL data from diverse populations of individuals with a variety of chronic diseases and demographic characteristics. Currently HHS monitors HRQOL in the United States by administering selected PROMIS and other HRQOL items on the Behavioral Risk Factors Surveillance System (BRFSS), the National Health and Nutrition Examination Survey (NHANES), and the National Health Interview Survey (NHIS).

The PROMIS item banks include more than 1,000 self-report questions covering multiple HRQOL domains that have undergone rigorous qualitative and quantitative evaluation by both patients and experts. A 10-item global HRQOL scale was developed to assess selected physical and mental health symptoms, including functioning and general health perceptions. The items were derived from HRQOL item banks which provide more precise indicators of domain-specific HRQOL. All items were tested in large and diverse samples. Individual items include fatigue, pain, emotional distress, and social activities. Most of the questions ask about a person's experience "in general" and assess self-reported symptoms within the last 7 days. The PROMIS measure provides an efficient assessment of HRQOL with minimal respondent burden and allows one to also estimate 2 summary measures of physical and mental health.

People with higher levels of well-being judge their life as going well. People feel very healthy and full of energy to take on their daily activities. People are satisfied, interested, and engaged with their lives. People experience a sense of accomplishment from their activities and judge their lives to be meaningful. People are more often content or cheerful than depressed or anxious. People get along with others and experience good social relationships. Personal factors, social circumstances, and community environments influence well-being.

Well-being considers the physical, mental, and social aspects of a person's life. Physical well-being relates to vigor and vitality, feeling very healthy and full of energy. Mental well-being includes being satisfied with one's life; balancing positive and negative emotions; accepting one's self; finding purpose and meaning in one's life; seeking personal growth, autonomy, and competence; believing one's life and circumstances are under one's control; and generally experiencing optimism. Social well-being involves providing and receiving quality support from family, friends, and others.

HRQOL and well-being also reflects individuals' assessment of the impact of their health and functional status on their participation in society. By measuring HRQOL through participation, quality of life is not directly equated to health or functional status but reflects, rather, the level of community integration or involvement, which is based on a person's level of participation, taking into account their health or functional status and the environment.

Underlying this participation measure is the principle that a person with a functional limitation — for example, vision loss, mobility difficulty, or intellectual disability — can live a long and productive life and enjoy a good quality of life. Poorer functional status can, and should not be, equated with poorer quality of life. Quality of life encompasses more than activities of daily living, health states, disease categories, or functional ability, "because it directs attention to the more complete social, psychological, and spiritual being." Social participation can be assessed through a determination of the degree to which people experience barriers to full participation because of their current health state and the environment.

Participation in society includes education, employment, and civic, social, and leisure activities, as well as family role participation. Participation is measured in the context of a person's current health state and within the person's current social and physical environments, thus capturing a more objective construct of the HRQOL concept.

Under this model, health state and the social and physical environment are defined as causal or background factors that impact HRQOL. Social participation and a sense of well-being are then outcome indicators that in turn reflect or define HRQOL.

HEALTHCARE-ASSOCIATED INFECTIONS (HAI)

HAIs are infections that patients get while receiving treatment for medical or surgical conditions. They are among the leading causes of preventable deaths in the United States and are associated with a substantial increase in health care costs each year.

HAIs occur in all types of care settings, including:

- Acute care within hospitals
- Same-day surgical centers
- Ambulatory outpatient care in health care clinics
- Long-term care facilities (e.g., nursing homes and rehabilitation facilities)

In hospitals, HAIs lead to extended hospital stays, contribute to increased medical costs, and are a significant cause of morbidity and mortality. Several other sources have been identified as major contributors to HAI-related illness and deaths in the National Action Plan to Prevent Healthcare-Associated Infections: Roadmap to Elimination. Nearly 3 out of every 4 HAIs in the acute care hospital setting are a result of 1 of the following 4 categories of infection, listed in order of prevalence:

Catheter-associated urinary tract infections

Surgical site infections

Bloodstream infections

Pneumonia

HAIs are the most common complication of hospital care. However, recent studies suggest that implementing existing prevention practices can lead to up to a 70 percent reduction in certain HAIs. The financial benefit of using these prevention practices is estimated to be $25.0 billion to $31.5 billion in medical cost savings.

Risk factors for HAIs can be grouped into three general categories:

- Medical procedures and antibiotic use
- Organizational factors
- Patient characteristics

The behaviors of health care providers and their interactions with the health care system also influence the rate of HAIs. Factors that lead to HAIs include:

- Use and maintenance of medical devices, such as catheters and ventilators
- Complications following surgical procedures

- Transmission between patients and health care workers

Other issues that increase the risk of HAIs are:

- Contaminated air conditioning systems
- Disproportionate nurse-to-patient ratio
- Physical layout of the health care facility (for example, open beds close together)

Studies have shown that proper education and training of health care workers increases compliance with and adoption of best practices to prevent HAIs. An example of a best practice by a health care provider is the careful use of antibiotics or antimicrobial drugs, as some can increase the patient's risk of HAIs.

Many efforts to prevent HAIs have focused on acute care settings. Increasingly, health care delivery, including complex procedures, is being shifted to outpatient settings, such as ambulatory surgical centers, end-stage renal disease facilities, and long-term care facilities. These settings often have limited capacity for oversight and infection control compared to hospital-based settings. Many HAIs in these settings are the result of poor basic infection-control practices. HAIs in outpatient settings happen because of:

- Improper sterilization and disinfection practices
- Reuse of syringes and needles
- Using single-use medication vials for multiple patients.

The National Action Plan to Prevent Healthcare-Associated Infections: Roadmap to Elimination contains strategies on preventing HAIs in non-acute care hospital settings and supports further research on how to identify and control HAIs in these settings and apply evidence-based approaches for reducing HAIs.

HEARING AND OTHER SENSORY OR COMMUNICATION DISORDERS

At least 1 in 6 Americans currently has a sensory or communication impairment or disorder. Even when they are temporary or mild, such disorders can affect physical and mental health. An impaired ability to communicate with others or maintain good balance can lead many people to:

- Feel socially isolated.
- Have unmet health needs.

- Have limited success in school or on the job.

An impaired sense of smell or taste can lead to poor nutrition or the inability to detect smoke, gas leaks, or foods that are unsafe to eat.

Communication and other sensory processes contribute to our overall health and well-being. Protecting these processes is critical, particularly for people whose age, race, ethnicity, gender, occupation, genetic background, or health status places them at increased risk. The Healthy People 2020 objectives are designed to ensure that all Americans, from birth through old age, will benefit from scientific advances in prevention, diagnosis, and treatment of hearing and other sensory or communication disorders. For example:

- One to 3 out of every 1,000 children is born with hearing loss. Through early diagnosis and intervention, these children can develop speech and language skills on schedule with their peers.
- Autism spectrum disorders, which often influence a child's ability to use language, affect 1 out of 110 8-year-old children. Researchers are investigating better ways to predict risk for autism in hopes of offering earlier treatment
- Obesity, diabetes, hypertension, malnutrition, Parkinson's disease, Alzheimer's disease, and multiple sclerosis are accompanied or signaled by chemosensory (smell and taste) problems. Diagnosis of chemosensory disorders may lead to earlier, more effective treatment of related diseases and conditions.
- Approximately 7.5 million people in the United States have trouble using their voices. People in occupations that stress the vocal cords, such as teaching and singing, may need preventive and rehabilitative services.

Substantial progress has been made in the development of alternative and augmentative communication devices that help people with severe disorders communicate.

Many factors influence the numbers of Americans who are diagnosed and treated for hearing and other sensory or communication disorders. A wide gap in overall health exists between people of higher and lower social and economic standings. For people of lower income, decreased access to routine and specialized health care adds to this disparity.

Another factor is the age at which a person is diagnosed or receives intervention, such as for infants born with hearing loss. Nearly all U.S. States participate in programs to screen newborns for hearing loss. These programs support early and appropriate intervention services that help improve children's social, emotional, cognitive, and academic growth.

Some individuals with hearing loss who could benefit from a hearing aid choose not to wear one due to the high cost or the perceived stigma of wearing an aid.

Unhealthy lifestyle choices, such as tobacco use or long-term exposure to loud noise without hearing protection, increase the prevalence and severity of hearing loss and other sensory and communication disorders.

Biological causes of hearing loss and other sensory or communication disorders include:

- Genetics
- Viral or bacterial infections
- Sensitivity to certain drugs or medications
- Injury
- Aging

Age may influence treatment options. For example, children as young as 12 months old with severe hearing loss are now receiving cochlear (inner-ear) implants.

As the Nation's population ages and survival rates for medically fragile infants and for people with severe injuries and acquired diseases improve, the prevalence of sensory and communication disorders is expected to rise.

Increases in blast exposure in combat situations have led to a dramatic rise in traumatic brain injury and ear damage in military personnel. These injuries have caused auditory disorders, such as hearing loss and tinnitus, and balance disorders, such as dizziness and vertigo. Noise-induced hearing loss may be reduced through the development of better ear-protection devices and emerging research into interventions that may protect or repair hair cells in the ear, which are key to the body's ability to hear.

Researchers are also identifying the genetic components of many disorders, which may lead to earlier and more accurate diagnosis, classification, and long-term clinical intervention. Research is adding to the understanding of co-occurring conditions and the way the presence of one disorder may lead to diagnosis and treatment of another, such as diagnosing Alzheimer's disease or Parkinson's disease through testing of olfactory (smell) function. In addition, hearing loss may be a largely unrecognized complication of diabetes, which suggests that people with diabetes should be screened for hearing loss.

HEART DISEASE AND STROKE

Heart disease is the leading cause of death in the United States. Stroke is the third leading cause of death in the United States. Together, heart disease and stroke are among the most widespread and costly health problems facing the Nation today, accounting for more than $500 billion in health care expenditures and related expenses in 2010 alone, according to the American Heart Foundation. Fortunately, they are also among the most preventable.

The leading modifiable (controllable) risk factors for heart disease and stroke are:

- High blood pressure
- High cholesterol
- Cigarette smoking
- Diabetes
- Poor diet and physical inactivity
- Overweight and obesity

Over time, these risk factors cause changes in the heart and blood vessels that can lead to heart attacks, heart failure, and strokes. It is critical to address risk factors early in life to prevent the potentially devastating complications of chronic cardiovascular disease.

Controlling risk factors for heart disease and stroke remains a challenge. High blood pressure and cholesterol are still major contributors to the national epidemic of cardiovascular disease. High blood pressure affects approximately 1 in 3 adults in the United States, and more than half of Americans with high blood pressure do not have it under control. High sodium intake is a known risk factor for high blood pressure and heart disease, yet about 90 percent of American adults exceed their recommendation for sodium intake.

The risk of Americans developing and dying from cardiovascular disease would be substantially reduced if major improvements were made across the U.S. population in diet and physical activity, control of high blood pressure and cholesterol, smoking cessation, and appropriate aspirin use.

Currently more than 1 in 3 adults (81.1 million) live with 1 or more types of cardiovascular disease. In addition to being the first and third leading causes of death, heart disease and stroke result in serious illness and disability, decreased quality of life, and hundreds of billions of dollars in economic loss every year.

The burden of cardiovascular disease is disproportionately distributed across the population. There are significant disparities in the following based on gender, age, race/ethnicity, geographic area, and socioeconomic status:

- Prevalence of risk factors
- Access to treatment
- Appropriate and timely treatment
- Treatment outcomes
- Mortality

Disease does not occur in isolation, and cardiovascular disease is no exception. Cardiovascular health is significantly influenced by the physical, social, and political environment, including:

- Maternal and child health
- Access to educational opportunities
- Availability of healthy foods, physical education, and extracurricular activities in schools
- Opportunities for physical activity, including access to safe and walkable communities
- Access to healthy foods
- Quality of working conditions and worksite health
- Availability of community support and resources
- Access to affordable, quality health care

No national system exists to collect data on how often cardiovascular events occur or recur, or how often they result in death. Similarly, there is inadequate tracking of quality indicators across the continuum of care, from risk factor prevention through treatment of acute events to posthospitalization and rehabilitation. New measures and tools are needed to monitor improvement in cardiovascular health over the next decade.

Other emerging issues in cardiovascular health include:

- Defining and measuring overall cardiovascular health.
- Assessing and communicating lifetime risk for cardiovascular disease.
- Addressing depression as a risk factor for and associated condition of heart disease and stroke.
- Examining cognitive impairment due to vascular disease.
- Dealing with substantial gaps in the cardiovascular surveillance system.

HIV

The HIV epidemic in the United States continues to be a major public health crisis. An estimated 1.1 million Americans are living with HIV, and 1 out of 5 people with HIV do not know they have it. HIV continues to spread, leading to about 56,000 new HIV infections each year.

In 2010, the White House released a National HIV/AIDS Strategy. The strategy includes 3 primary goals:

Reducing the number of people who become infected with HIV.

Increasing access to care and improving health outcomes for people living with HIV.

Reducing HIV-related health disparities.

HIV is a preventable disease. Effective HIV prevention interventions have been proven to reduce HIV transmission. People who get tested for HIV and learn that they are infected can make significant behavior changes to improve their health and reduce the risk of transmitting HIV to their sex or drug-using partners. More than 50 percent of new HIV infections3 occur as a result of the 21 percent of people who have HIV but do not know it.

In the era of increasingly effective treatments for HIV, people with HIV are living longer, healthier, and more productive lives. Deaths from HIV infection have greatly declined in the United States since the 1990s. As the number of people living with HIV grows, it will be more important than ever to increase national HIV prevention and health care programs.

However, there are still gender, race, and ethnicity disparities in new HIV infections.

- Nearly 75 percent of new HIV infections occur in men.
- More than half occur in gay and bisexual men, regardless of race or ethnicity.
- Forty-five percent of new HIV infections occur in African Americans, 35 percent in whites, and 17 percent in Hispanics.

Improving access to quality health care for populations disproportionately affected by HIV, such as persons of color and gay and bisexual men, is a fundamental public health strategy for HIV prevention. People getting care for HIV can receive:

- Antiretroviral therapy
- Screening and treatment for other diseases (such as sexually transmitted infections)
- HIV prevention interventions

- Mental health services
- Other health services

As the number of people living with HIV increases and more people become aware of their HIV status, prevention strategies that are targeted specifically for HIV-infected people are becoming more important. Prevention work with people living with HIV focuses on:

- Linking to and staying in treatment.
- Increasing the availability of ongoing HIV prevention interventions.
- Providing prevention services for their partners.

It is also important to foster wider availability of comprehensive services for people living with HIV and their partners through partnerships among health departments, community-based organizations, and health care and social service providers.

Public perception in the United States about the seriousness of the HIV epidemic has declined in recent years. There is evidence that risky behaviors may be increasing among uninfected people, especially gay and bisexual men. Ongoing media and social campaigns for the general public and HIV prevention interventions for uninfected persons who engage in risky behaviors are critical.

IMMUNIZATION AND INFECTIOUS DISEASES

The increase in life expectancy during the 20th century is largely due to improvements in child survival; this increase is associated with reductions in infectious disease mortality, due largely to immunization. However, infectious diseases remain a major cause of illness, disability, and death. Immunization recommendations in the United States currently target 17 vaccine-preventable diseases across the lifespan.

HHS goals for immunization and infectious diseases are rooted in evidence-based clinical and community activities and services for the prevention and treatment of infectious diseases. Objectives new to Healthy People 2020 focus on technological advancements and ensuring that States, local public health departments, and nongovernmental organizations are strong partners in the Nation's attempt to control the spread of infectious diseases. These objectives reflect a more mobile society and the fact that diseases do not stop at geopolitical borders. Awareness of disease and completing prevention and treatment courses remain essential components for reducing infectious disease transmission.

People in the United States continue to get diseases that are vaccine preventable. Viral hepatitis, influenza, and tuberculosis (TB) remain among the leading causes of illness and death in the United States and account for substantial spending on the related consequences of infection.

The infectious disease public health infrastructure, which carries out disease surveillance at the Federal, State, and local levels, is an essential tool in the fight against newly emerging and re-emerging infectious diseases. Other important defenses against infectious diseases include:

- Proper use of vaccines
- Antibiotics
- Screening and testing guidelines
- Scientific improvements in the diagnosis of infectious disease-related health concerns

Vaccines are among the most cost-effective clinical preventive services and are a core component of any preventive services package. Childhood immunization programs provide a very high return on investment. For example, for each birth cohort vaccinated with the routine immunization schedule (this includes DTap, Td, Hib, Polio, MMR, Hep B, and varicella vaccines), society:

- Saves 33,000 lives.
- Prevents 14 million cases of disease.
- Reduces direct health care costs by $9.9 billion.
- Saves $33.4 billion in indirect costs.

Despite progress, approximately 42,000 adults and 300 children in the United States die each year from vaccine-preventable diseases. Communities with pockets of unvaccinated and undervaccinated populations are at increased risk for outbreaks of vaccine-preventable diseases. In 2008, imported measles resulted in 140 reported cases—nearly a 3-fold increase over the previous year. The emergence of new or replacement strains of vaccine-preventable disease can result in a significant increase in serious illnesses and death.

The Nation's public health goals focus on reducing illness, hospitalization, and death from vaccine-preventable diseases and other infectious diseases; expanding surveillance is crucial to those ends. Further efforts to improve disease surveillance will allow for earlier detection of the emergence and spread of diseases. Increased surveillance will save lives by allowing the maximum time possible for public health responses, including vaccine production and development of evidence-based recommendations on disease prevention and control. Surveillance enables rapid information sharing and facilitates the timely identification of people in need of immediate treatment. Increasing laboratory capacity is essential for these efforts.

Acute respiratory infections, including pneumonia and influenza, are the 8th leading cause of death in the United States, accounting for 56,000 deaths annually. Pneumonia mortality in children fell by 97 percent in the last century, but respiratory infectious diseases continue to be leading causes of pediatric hospitalization and outpatient visits in the United States. On average, influenza leads to more than 200,000 hospitalizations and 36,000 deaths each year. The 2009 H1N1 influenza pandemic caused an estimated 270,000 hospitalizations and 12,270 deaths (1,270 of which were of people younger than age 18) between April 2009 and March 2010.

Viral hepatitis and TB can be prevented, yet health care systems often do not make the best use of their available resources to support prevention efforts. Because the U.S. health care system focuses on treatment of illnesses, rather than health promotion, patients do not always receive information about prevention and healthy lifestyles. This includes advancing effective and evidence-based viral hepatitis and TB prevention priorities and interventions.

In the coming decade, the United States will continue to face new and emerging issues in the area of immunization and infectious diseases. The public health infrastructure must be capable of responding to emerging threats. State-of-the-art technology and highly skilled professionals need to be in place to provide rapid response to the threat of epidemics. A coordinated strategy is necessary to understand, detect, control, and prevent infectious diseases. Below are some specific emerging issues:

- Providing culturally appropriate preventive health care is an immediate responsibility that will grow over the decade. As the demographics of the population continue to shift, public health and health care systems will need to expand their capacity to protect the growing needs of a diverse and aging population.
- New infectious agents and diseases continue to be detected. Infectious diseases must be looked at in a global context due to increasing:
  - International travel and trade
  - Migration
  - Importation of foods and agricultural practices

~ Threats of bioterrorism

- Inappropriate use of antibiotics and environmental changes multiply the potential for worldwide epidemics of all types of infectious diseases.

Infectious diseases are a critical public health, humanitarian, and security concern; coordinated efforts will protect people across the Nation and around the world.

INJURY AND VIOLENCE PREVENTION

Injuries and violence are widespread in society. Both unintentional injuries and those caused by acts of violence are among the top 15 killers for Americans of all ages. Many people accept them as "accidents," "acts of fate," or as "part of life." However, most events resulting in injury, disability, or death are predictable and preventable.

Injuries are the leading cause of death for Americans ages 1 to 44, and a leading cause of disability for all ages, regardless of sex, race/ethnicity, or socioeconomic status. More than 180,000 people die from injuries each year, and approximately 1 in 10 sustains a nonfatal injury serious enough to be treated in a hospital emergency department.

Beyond their immediate health consequences, injuries and violence have a significant impact on the well-being of Americans by contributing to:

- Premature death
- Disability
- Poor mental health
- High medical costs
- Lost productivity

The effects of injuries and violence extend beyond the injured person or victim of violence to family members, friends, coworkers, employers, and communities.

Numerous determinants (factors) can affect the risk of unintentional injury and violence.

The choices people make about individual behaviors, such as alcohol use or risk-taking, can increase injuries. The physical environment, both in the home and community, can affect the rate of injuries related to falls, fires and burns, road traffic injuries, drowning, and violence. Access to health services, such as systems created for injury-related care, ranging from prehospital and acute care to rehabilitation, can reduce the consequences of injuries, including death and long-term disability.

The social environment has a notable influence on the risk for injury and violence through:

- Individual social experiences (for example, social norms, education, victimization history)
- Social relationships (for example, parental monitoring and supervision of youth, peer group associations, family interactions)
- Community environment (for example, cohesion in schools, neighborhoods, and communities)
- Societal-level factors (for example, cultural beliefs, attitudes, incentives and disincentives, laws and regulations)

Interventions that address these social and physical factors have the potential to prevent unintentional injuries and violence. Efforts to prevent unintentional injury may focus on:

- Modifications of the environment
- Improvements in product safety
- Legislation and enforcement
- Education and behavior change
- Technology and engineering

Efforts to prevent violence may focus on:

- Changing social norms about the acceptability of violence
- Improving problem-solving skills (for example, parenting, conflict resolution, coping)
- Changing policies to address the social and economic conditions that often give rise to violence

There are several emerging issues in injury and violence prevention that need further research, analysis, and monitoring. For unintentional injuries, there is a need to better understand the trends, causes, and prevention strategies for:

- Motor vehicle crashes due to distracted driving
- Injuries related to recreational activities

In the area of violence, there is a need to better understand the trends, causes, and prevention strategies related to:

- Bullying, dating violence, and sexual violence among youth
- Elder maltreatment, particularly with respect to quantifying and understanding the problem

LESBIAN, GAY, BISEXUAL, AND TRANSGENDER (LGBT) HEALTH

LGBT individuals encompass all races and ethnicities, religions, and social classes. Sexual orientation and gender identity questions are not asked on most national or State surveys, making it difficult to estimate the number of LGBT individuals and their health needs.

Research suggests that LGBT individuals face health disparities linked to societal stigma, discrimination, and denial of their civil and human rights. Discrimination against LGBT persons has been associated with high rates of psychiatric disorders, substance abuse, and suicide. Experiences of violence and victimization are frequent for LGBT individuals, and have long-lasting effects on the individual and the community. Personal, family, and social acceptance of sexual orientation and gender identity affects the mental health and personal safety of LGBT individuals.

More research is needed to document, understand, and address the environmental factors that contribute to health disparities in the LGBT community.

Eliminating LGBT health disparities and enhancing efforts to improve LGBT health are necessary to ensure that LGBT individuals can lead long, healthy lives. The many benefits of addressing health concerns and reducing disparities include:

- Reductions in disease transmission and progression
- Increased mental and physical well-being
- Reduced health care costs
- Increased longevity

Efforts to improve LGBT health include:

- Curbing human immunodeficiency virus (HIV)/sexually transmitted diseases (STDs) with interventions that work.
- Implementing antibullying policies in schools.
- Providing supportive social services to reduce suicide and homelessness risk among youth.
- Appropriately inquiring about and being supportive of a patient's sexual orientation to enhance the patient-provider interaction and regular use of care.
- Providing medical students with access to LGBT patients to increase provision of culturally competent care.

Efforts to address health disparities among LGBT persons include:

- Expansion of domestic partner health insurance coverage

- Establishment of LGBT health centers
- Dissemination of effective HIV/STD interventions

Understanding LGBT health starts with understanding the history of oppression and discrimination that these communities have faced. For example, in part because bars and clubs were often the only safe places where LGBT individuals could gather, alcohol abuse has been an ongoing problem. Social determinants affecting the health of LGBT individuals largely relate to oppression and discrimination. Examples include:

- Legal discrimination in access to health insurance, employment, housing, marriage, adoption, and retirement benefits
- Lack of laws protecting against bullying in schools
- Lack of social programs targeted to and/or appropriate for LGBT youth, adults, and elders
- Shortage of health care providers who are knowledgeable and culturally competent in LGBT health

The physical environment that contributes to healthy LGBT individuals includes:

- Safe schools, neighborhoods, and housing
- Access to recreational facilities and activities
- Availability of safe meeting places
- Access to health services

LGBT health requires specific attention from health care and public health professionals to address a number of disparities, including:

- LGBT youth are 2 to 3 times more likely to attempt suicide.
- LGBT youth are more likely to be homeless.
- Lesbians are less likely to get preventive services for cancer.
- Gay men are at higher risk of HIV and other STDs, especially among communities of color
- Lesbians and bisexual females are more likely to be overweight or obese.
- Transgender individuals have a high prevalence of HIV/STDs, victimization, mental health issues, and suicide and are less likely to have health insurance than heterosexual or LGB individuals.
- Elderly LGBT individuals face additional barriers to health because of isolation and a lack of social services and culturally competent providers.
- LGBT populations have the highest rates of tobacco, alcohol, and other drug use.

A number of issues will need to continue to be evaluated and addressed over the coming decade, including:

- Prevention of violence and homicide toward the LGB community, and especially the transgender population
- Nationally representative data on LGBT Americans
- Resiliency in LGBT communities
- LGBT parenting issues throughout the life course
- Elder health and well-being
- Exploration of sexual/gender identity among youth
- Need for a LGBT wellness model
- Recognition of transgender health needs as medically necessary

MATERNAL, INFANT, AND CHILD HEALTH

Improving the well-being of mothers, infants, and children is an important public health goal for the United States. Their well-being determines the health of the next generation and can help predict future public health challenges for families, communities, and the health care system. The objectives of the Maternal, Infant, and Child Health topic area address a wide range of conditions, health behaviors, and health systems indicators that affect the health, wellness, and quality of life of women, children, and families.

Pregnancy can provide an opportunity to identify existing health risks in women and to prevent future health problems for women and their children. These health risks may include:

- Hypertension and heart disease
- Diabetes
- Depression
- Genetic conditions
- Sexually transmitted diseases (STDs)
- Tobacco use and alcohol abuse
- Inadequate nutrition
- Unhealthy weight

The risk of maternal and infant mortality and pregnancy-related complications can be reduced by increasing access to quality preconception (before pregnancy) and interconception (between pregnancies) care. Moreover, healthy birth outcomes and early identification and treatment of health conditions among infants can prevent death or disability and enable children to reach their full potential.

Many factors can affect pregnancy and childbirth, including:
- Preconception health status
- Age
- Access to appropriate preconception and interconception health care
- Poverty

Infant and child health are similarly influenced by socio-demographic factors, such as family income, but are also linked to the physical and mental health of parents and caregivers. There are racial and ethnic disparities in mortality and morbidity for mothers and children, particularly for African Americans. These differences are likely the result of many factors.

These include pre-pregnancy health behaviors and health status, which are influenced by a variety of environmental and social factors such as access to health care and chronic stress.

Common barriers to a healthy pregnancy and birth include lack of access to appropriate health care before and during pregnancy. In addition, environmental factors can shape a woman's overall health status before, during, and after pregnancy by:
- Affecting her health directly.
- Affecting her ability to engage in healthy behaviors.

The social determinants that influence maternal health also affect pregnancy outcomes and infant health. Racial and ethnic disparities in infant mortality exist, particularly for African American infants. Child health status varies by both race and ethnicity, as well as by family income and related factors, including educational attainment among household members and health insurance coverage.

The cognitive and physical development of infants and children is influenced by the health, nutrition, and behaviors of their mothers during pregnancy and early childhood. Breast milk is widely acknowledged to be the most complete form of nutrition for most infants, with a range of benefits for their health, growth, immunity, and development. Furthermore, children reared in safe and nurturing families and neighborhoods, free from maltreatment and other social adversities, are more likely to have better outcomes as adults.

Recent efforts to address persistent disparities in maternal, infant, and child health have employed a "life course" perspective to health promotion and disease prevention. At the start of the decade, fewer than half of all pregnancies are planned. Unintended pregnancy is associated with a host of public health concerns. In response, preconception health initiatives have been aimed at improving the health of a woman before she becomes pregnant through a variety of evidence-based interventions.

The life course perspective also supports the examination of quality of life, including the challenges of male and female fertility. An estimated 7.3 million American women ages 15 to 44 have received infertility services (including counseling and diagnosis) in their lifetime. Infertility is an area where health disparities are large, particularly among African American women, and may only continue to increase as childbearing practices change over time.

MEDICAL PRODUCT SAFETY

The Medical Product Safety objectives for 2020 focus on overall improvement of patient treatment and appropriate use of medical products. Medical products include drugs, biological products, and medical devices. These objectives reflect strong scientific support for safe use of medical products, which promotes better health among Americans.

Increasing appropriate use and monitoring adverse effects of medical products will:

- Decrease adverse events and harmful reactions by focusing safety efforts.
- Improve the overall effectiveness of treatment by reducing harm from medical products.
- Further personalize medical treatment.

Many factors influence the safety of medical products and their effects on patients. These factors include:

- A patient's genetic make-up and physiological condition
- Drug composition (ingredients), manufacturing, and labeling
- Appropriate use
- Monitoring for adverse effects

Incorrect use and inadequate monitoring of many medical products can cause adverse effects. For this reason, greater focus and emphasis on the safe use of such products is critical. Successfully reducing adverse events that result from medical products will improve overall treatment and increase the number of patients who benefit from medical products.

An important focus for the improvement of medical product safety is the expanded use of health information technology. The U.S. Department of Health and Human Services is coordinating efforts to develop a national health information technology infrastructure that would include electronic medical records, digital prescribing programs, and electronic decision-support programs. The system is intended to improve health care quality and patient safety by:

- Reducing medical errors.
- Improving communication to better inform and empower consumers.
- Enhancing the capacity of post-market surveillance to promptly and efficiently detect previously unknown problems with medical products.

Continued and innovative efforts are necessary to improve medical product safety and to meet the objectives for 2020.

MENTAL HEALTH AND MENTAL DISORDERS

Mental health is a state of successful performance of mental function, resulting in productive activities, fulfilling relationships with other people, and the ability to adapt to change and to cope with challenges. Mental health is essential to personal well-being, family and interpersonal relationships, and the ability to contribute to community or society.

Mental disorders are health conditions that are characterized by alterations in thinking, mood, and/or behavior that are associated with distress and/or impaired functioning. Mental disorders contribute to a host of problems that may include disability, pain, or death.

Mental illness is the term that refers collectively to all diagnosable mental disorders.

Mental disorders are among the most common causes of disability. The resulting disease burden of mental illness is among the highest of all diseases. According to the National Institute of Mental Health (NIMH), in any given year, an estimated 13 million American adults (approximately 1 in 17) have a seriously debilitating mental illness.

Mental health disorders are the leading cause of disability in the United States and Canada, accounting for 25 percent of all years of life lost to disability and premature mortality. Moreover, suicide is the 11th leading cause of death in the United States, accounting for the deaths of approximately 30,000 Americans each year.

Mental health and physical health are closely connected. Mental health plays a major role in people's ability to maintain good physical health. Mental illnesses, such as depression and anxiety, affect people's ability to participate in health-promoting behaviors. In turn, problems with physical health, such as chronic diseases, can have a serious impact on mental health and decrease a person's ability to participate in treatment and recovery.

The existing model for understanding mental health and mental disorders emphasizes the interaction of social, environmental, and genetic factors throughout the lifespan. In behavioral health, researchers identify:

- Risk factors, which predispose individuals to mental illness
- Protective factors, which protect them from developing mental disorders

Researchers now know that the prevention of mental, emotional, and behavioral (MEB) disorders is inherently interdisciplinary and draws on a variety of different strategies. Over the past 20 years, research on the prevention of mental disorders has progressed. The understanding of how the brain functions under normal conditions and in response to stressors, combined with knowledge of how the brain develops over time, has been essential to that progress. The major areas of progress include evidence that:

- MEB disorders are common and begin early in life.
- The greatest opportunity for prevention is among young people.
- There are multiyear effects of multiple preventive interventions on reducing substance abuse, conduct disorder, antisocial behavior, aggression, and child maltreatment.
- The incidence of depression among pregnant women and adolescents can be reduced.

School-based violence prevention can reduce the base rate of aggressive problems in an average school by 25 to 33 percent.

There are potential indicated preventive interventions for schizophrenia.

Improving family functioning and positive parenting can have positive outcomes on mental health and can reduce poverty-related risk.

School-based preventive interventions aimed at improving social and emotional outcomes can also improve academic outcomes.

Interventions targeting families dealing with adversities, such as parental depression or divorce, can be effective in reducing risk for depression among children and increasing effective parenting.

Some preventive interventions have benefits that exceed costs, with the available evidence strongest for early childhood interventions.

Implementation is complex, and it is important that interventions be relevant to the target audiences.

The progress identified above has led to a stronger understanding of the importance of protective factors. A 2009 Institute of Medicine (IOM) report advocates for multidisciplinary prevention strategies at the community level that support the development of children in healthy social environments. In addition to advancements in the prevention of mental disorders, there continues to be steady progress in treating mental disorders as new drugs and stronger evidence-based outcomes become available.

New mental health issues have emerged among some special populations, such as:

- Veterans who have experienced physical and mental trauma
- People in communities with large-scale psychological trauma caused by natural disasters
- Older adults, as the understanding and treatment of dementia and mood disorders continues to improve

As the Federal Government begins to implement health reform legislation, it will give attention to providing services for individuals with mental illness and substance use disorders, including new opportunities for access to and coverage for treatment and prevention services.

NUTRITION AND WEIGHT STATUS

There is strong science supporting the health benefits of eating a healthful diet and maintaining a healthy body weight. Efforts to change diet and weight should address individual behaviors, as well as the policies and environments that support these behaviors in settings such as schools, worksites, health care organizations, and communities. The goal of promoting healthful diets and healthy weight encompasses increasing household food security and eliminating hunger.

Americans with a healthful diet:

- Consume a variety of nutrient-dense foods within and across the food groups, especially whole grains, fruits, vegetables, low-fat or fat-free milk or milk products, and lean meats and other protein sources.

- Limit the intake of saturated and trans fats, cholesterol, added sugars, sodium (salt), and alcohol.
- Limit caloric intake to meet caloric needs.

All Americans should avoid unhealthy weight gain, and those whose weight is too high may also need to lose weight.

Diet and body weight are related to health status. Good nutrition is important to the growth and development of children. A healthful diet also helps Americans reduce their risks for many health conditions, including:

- Overweight and obesity
- Malnutrition
- Iron-deficiency anemia
- Heart disease
- High blood pressure
- Dyslipidemia (poor lipid profiles)
- Type 2 diabetes
- Osteoporosis
- Oral disease
- Constipation
- Diverticular disease
- Some cancers

Individuals who are at a healthy weight are less likely to:

- Develop chronic disease risk factors, such as high blood pressure and dyslipidemia.
- Develop chronic diseases, such as type 2 diabetes, heart disease, osteoarthritis, and some cancers.
- Experience complications during pregnancy.

Die at an earlier age.

Diet reflects the variety of foods and beverages consumed over time and in settings such as worksites, schools, restaurants, and the home. Interventions to support a healthier diet can help ensure that:

- Individuals have the knowledge and skills to make healthier choices.
- Healthier options are available and affordable.

Demographic characteristics of those with a more healthful diet vary with the nutrient or food studied. However, most Americans need to improve some aspect of their diet.

Social factors thought to influence diet include:

- Knowledge and attitudes
- Skills
- Social support

- Societal and cultural norms
- Food and agricultural policies
- Food assistance programs
- Economic price systems

Access to and availability of healthier foods can help people follow healthful diets. For example, better access to retail venues that sell healthier options may have a positive impact on a person's diet; these venues may be less available in low-income or rural neighborhoods.

The places where people eat appear to influence their diet. For example, foods eaten away from home often have more calories and are of lower nutritional quality than foods prepared at home. Marketing also influences people's—particularly children's—food choices.

Because weight is influenced by energy (calories) consumed and expended, interventions to improve weight can support changes in diet or physical activity. They can help change individuals' knowledge and skills, reduce exposure to foods low in nutritional value and high in calories, or increase opportunities for physical activity. Interventions can help prevent unhealthy weight gain or facilitate weight loss among obese people. They can be delivered in multiple settings, including health care settings, worksites, or schools.

The social and physical factors affecting diet and physical activity (see Physical Activity topic area) may also have an impact on weight.

Obesity is a problem throughout the population. However, among adults, the prevalence is highest for middle-aged people and for non-Hispanic black and Mexican American women. Among children and adolescents, the prevalence of obesity is highest among older and Mexican American children and non-Hispanic black girls. The association of income with obesity varies by age, gender, and race/ethnicity.

As new and innovative policy and environmental interventions to support diet and physical activity are implemented, it will be important to identify which are most effective. A better understanding of how to prevent unhealthy weight gain is also needed.

OCCUPATIONAL SAFETY AND HEALTH

Work-related illnesses and injuries include any illness or injury incurred by an employee engaged in work-related activities while on or off the worksite.

Workplace settings vary widely in size, sector, design, location, work processes, workplace culture, and resources. In addition, workers themselves are different in terms of age, gender, training, education, cultural background, health practices, and access to preventive health care. This translates to great diversity in the safety and health risks for each industry sector and the need for tailored interventions.

The National Occupational Research Agenda (NORA) was established by the Centers for Disease Control and Prevention (CDC) National Institute for Occupational Safety and Health (NIOSH) and its partners to stimulate research and improve workplace practices. Now in its second decade (2006–2016), NORA focuses on occupational safety and health in 10 sectors:

- Agriculture, Forestry, and Fishing
- Construction
- Health Care and Social Assistance
- Manufacturing
- Mining
- Oil and Gas Extraction
- Public Safety
- Services
- Transportation, Warehousing, and Utilities
- Wholesale and Retail Trade

The U.S. civilian workforce employed approximately 140 million people in 2009, according to the U.S. Department of Labor, Bureau of Labor Statistics. These workers spend a quarter of their lifetime, and up to half of their waking lives, at work or commuting. Despite improvements in occupational safety and health over the last several decades, workers continue to suffer work-related deaths, injuries, and illnesses. The workplace, therefore, provides a unique forum for public health action.

Work is one of the most important determinants of a person's health. However, addressing occupational safety and health poses numerous challenges.

The workforce, like the U.S. population at large, is becoming increasingly diverse. These demographic changes result in new safety and health issues. For example, some workers—such as racial and ethnic minorities, recent immigrants, younger and older workers, workers with genetic susceptibility, and workers with disabilities—are more likely to have increased risks of work-related diseases and injuries.

Workplaces are rapidly evolving as jobs in the current economy continue to shift from manufacturing to services.

Major changes are also occurring in the way work is organized. Longer hours, compressed work weeks, shift work, reduced job security, and part-time and temporary work are realities of the modern workplace and are increasingly affecting the health and lives of workers.

Finally, the new chemicals, materials, processes, and equipment that are being developed at an ever-accelerating pace pose emerging risks to occupational health.

Despite these challenges, the Nation is poised to make significant improvements over the coming decade in the quality of life for all working people. Occupational safety and health research has led to many changes in workplaces and work processes that prevent injuries, illnesses, and deaths in workers. Ongoing research seeks to identify new and better ways to improve the health and safety of workers and to identify and address emerging hazards. In addition, scientists and partners are working together to translate and transfer research findings, technologies, and information into highly effective interventions and products that can be readily integrated into the workplace, resulting in more immediate improvements in the lives of workers.

Other new approaches to occupational safety and health include eliminating workplace hazards that result from design flaws and integrating the protection of the worker in the workplace with the promotion of a healthy lifestyle at home.

Although improvements in occupational safety and health surveillance are ongoing, there are several emerging areas in which national data systems are not yet available or merit further research. For example, there are recognized data gaps in understanding the safety and health effects of exposure to nanoparticles—the ultrafine, manipulated particles used in many industries. Nanoparticles have numerous applications to areas ranging from medicine to manufacturing. Nanotechnology is anticipated to increase to a trillion-dollar industry employing millions of workers worldwide within the next decade. NIOSH and its partners are conducting research to better understand the health effects of nanotechnology, establish an evidence base on risks and controls, and develop appropriate guidance.

OLDER ADULTS

Older adults are among the fastest growing age groups, and the first "baby boomers" (adults born between 1946 and 1964) turned 65 in 2011. More than 37 million people in this group (60 percent) will manage more than 1 chronic condition by 2030.

Older adults are at high risk for developing chronic illnesses and related disabilities. These chronic conditions include:

- Diabetes mellitus
- Arthritis
- Congestive heart failure
- Dementia

Many experience hospitalizations, nursing home admissions, and low-quality care. They also may lose the ability to live independently at home. Chronic conditions are the leading cause of death among older adults.

Preventive health services are valuable for maintaining the quality of life and wellness of older adults. In fact, the Patient Protection and Affordable Care Act of 2010 includes provisions related to relevant Medicare services. However, preventive services are underused, especially among certain racial and ethnic groups.

Ensuring quality health care for older adults is difficult, but the Centers for Medicare & Medicaid Services (CMS) has programs designed to improve physician, hospital, and nursing home care, among others.

Older adults use many health care services, have complex conditions, and require professional expertise that meets their needs. Most providers receive some type of training on aging, but the percentage of those who actually specialize in this area is small. More certified specialists are needed to meet the needs of this group.

Through programs that address chronic illnesses, Federal Government agencies are improving the quality of life for older adults. To combat existing health disparities, many of these programs target minorities and underserved populations.

The ability to complete basic daily activities may decrease if illness, chronic disease, or injury limit physical or mental abilities of older adults. These limitations make it hard for older adults to remain at home. Early prevention and physical activity can help prevent such declines. Unfortunately, less than 20 percent of older adults engage in enough physical activity, and fewer do strength training. Minority populations often have lower rates of physical activity.

Most older adults want to remain in their communities as long as possible. Unfortunately, when they acquire disabilities, there is often not enough support available to help them. States that invest in such services show lower rates of growth in long-term care expenditures.

Each year, 1 out of 3 older adults falls. Falls often cause severe disability among survivors. Injuries from falls lead to:

- Fear of falling
- Sedentary behavior
- Impaired function
- Lower quality of life

Falls are the leading cause of death due to unintentional injury among older adults; deaths and injuries can be prevented by addressing risk factors.

Caregivers for older adults living at home are typically unpaid family members. Caregiver stress often results in unnecessary nursing home placement. One to 2 million older adults in the United States are injured or mistreated by a loved one or a caregiver. A measure of elder abuse has been added to encourage data collection on this issue.

Many factors affect the health, function, and quality of life of older adults. Behaviors such as participation in physical activity, self-management of chronic diseases, or use of preventive health services can improve health outcomes.

Housing and transportation services affect the ability of older adults to access care. People from minority populations tend to be in poorer health and use health care less often than people from nonminority populations.

The quality of the health and social services available to older adults and their caregivers affects their ability to manage chronic conditions and long-term care needs effectively.

Emerging issues for improving the health of older adults include efforts to:

- Coordinate care.
- Help older adults manage their own care.
- Establish quality measures.
- Identify minimum levels of training for people who care for older adults.
- Research and analyze appropriate training to equip providers with the tools they need to meet the needs of older adults.

There is growing recognition that data sources are limited for certain subpopulations of older adults, including the aging lesbian, gay, bisexual, and transgender populations. Research for these groups will inform future health and policy initiatives.

ORAL HEALTH

The health of the mouth and surrounding craniofacial (skull and face) structures is central to a person's overall health and well-being. Oral and craniofacial diseases and conditions include:

- Dental caries (tooth decay)
- Periodontal (gum) diseases
- Cleft lip and palate
- Oral and facial pain
- Oral and pharyngeal (mouth and throat) cancers

The significant improvement in the oral health of Americans over the past 50 years is a public health success story. Most of the gains are a result of effective prevention and treatment efforts. One major success is community water fluoridation, which now benefits about 7 out of 10 Americans who get water through public water systems.

However, some Americans do not have access to preventive programs. People who have the least access to preventive services and dental treatment have greater rates of oral diseases. A person's ability to access oral health care is associated with factors such as education level, income, race, and ethnicity.

There is a need to:

- Increase awareness of the importance of oral health to overall health and well-being.
- Increase acceptance and adoption of effective preventive interventions.
- Reduce disparities in access to effective preventive and dental treatment services.

Oral health is essential to overall health. Good oral health improves a person's ability to speak, smile, smell, taste, touch, chew, swallow, and make facial expressions to show feelings and emotions. However, oral diseases, from cavities to oral cancer, cause pain and disability for many Americans.

Good self-care, such as brushing with fluoride toothpaste, daily flossing, and professional treatment, is key to good oral health. Health behaviors that can lead to poor oral health include:

- Tobacco use
- Excessive alcohol use
- Poor dietary choices

Barriers that can limit a person's use of preventive interventions and treatments include:

- Limited access to and availability of dental services
- Lack of awareness of the need for care
- Cost
- Fear of dental procedures

There are also social determinants that affect oral health. In general, people with lower levels of education and income, and people from specific racial/ethnic groups, have higher rates of disease. People with disabilities and other health conditions, like diabetes, are more likely to have poor oral health.

Community water fluoridation and school-based dental sealant programs are two leading evidence-based interventions to prevent tooth decay. Community water fluoridation is the most effective way to deliver the benefits of fluoride to a community. Studies show that it prevents tooth decay by 18 to 40 percent. School-based dental sealant programs, which focus on sealing permanent molar teeth, usually target schools that serve children from low-income families. Dental sealants can prevent up to 60 percent of tooth decay in the treated teeth.

Major improvements have occurred in the Nation's oral health, but some challenges remain and new concerns have emerged. One important emerging oral health issue is the increase of tooth decay in preschool children. A recent Centers for Disease Control and Prevention (CDC) publication reported that, over the past decade, dental caries (tooth decay) in children ages 2 to 5 have increased.

Lack of access to dental care for all ages remains a public health challenge. This issue was highlighted in a 2008 Government Accountability Office (GAO) report that described difficulties in accessing dental care for low-income children. In addition, the Institute of Medicine (IOM) has convened an expert panel to evaluate factors that influence access to dental care.

Potential strategies to address these issues include:

- Implementing and evaluating activities that have an impact on health behavior.
- Promoting interventions to reduce tooth decay, such as dental sealants and fluoride use.
- Evaluating and improving methods of monitoring oral diseases and conditions.
- Increasing the capacity of State dental health programs to provide preventive oral health services.
- Increasing the number of community health centers with an oral health component.

PHYSICAL ACTIVITY

Released in 2008, the Physical Activity Guidelines for Americans (PAG) is the first-ever publication of national guidelines for physical activity. Regular physical activity includes participation in moderate and vigorous physical activities and muscle-strengthening activities.

More than 80 percent of adults do not meet the guidelines for both aerobic and muscle-strengthening activities. Similarly, more than 80 percent of adolescents do not do enough aerobic physical activity to meet the guidelines for youth. A multidisciplinary approach is critical to increasing the levels of physical activity and improving health in the United States.

Regular physical activity can improve the health and quality of life of Americans of all ages, regardless of the presence of a chronic disease or disability. Among adults and older adults, physical activity can lower the risk of:
- Early death
- Coronary heart disease
- Stroke
- High blood pressure
- Type 2 diabetes
- Breast and colon cancer
- Falls
- Depression

Among children and adolescents, physical activity can:
- Improve bone health.

- Improve cardiorespiratory and muscular fitness.
- Decrease levels of body fat.
- Reduce symptoms of depression.

For people who are inactive, even small increases in physical activity are associated with health benefits.

Personal, social, economic, and environmental factors all play a role in physical activity levels among youth, adults, and older adults. Understanding the barriers to and facilitators of physical activity is important to ensure the effectiveness of interventions and other actions to improve levels of physical activity.

Factors positively associated with adult physical activity include:
- Postsecondary education
- Higher income
- Enjoyment of exercise
- Expectation of benefits
- Belief in ability to exercise (self-efficacy)
- History of activity in adulthood
- Social support from peers, family, or spouse
- Access to and satisfaction with facilities
- Enjoyable scenery
- Safe neighborhoods

Factors negatively associated with adult physical activity include:
- Advancing age
- Low income
- Lack of time
- Low motivation
- Rural residency
- Perception of great effort needed for exercise
- Overweight or obesity
- Perception of poor health
- Being disabled

Older adults may have additional factors that keep them from being physically active, including lack of social support, lack of transportation to facilities, fear of injury, and cost of programs. Among children ages 4 to 12, the following factors have a positive association with physical activity:
- Gender (boys)
- Belief in ability to be active (self-efficacy)
- Parental support

Among adolescents ages 13 to 18, the following factors have a positive association with physical activity:

- Parental education
- Gender (boys)
- Personal goals
- Physical education/school sports
- Belief in ability to be active (self-efficacy)
- Support of friends and family

Environmental influences positively associated with physical activity among children and adolescents include:

- Presence of sidewalks
- Having a destination/walking to a particular place
- Access to public transportation
- Low traffic density
- Access to neighborhood or school play area and/or recreational equipment6

People with disabilities may be less likely to participate in physical activity due to physical, emotional, and psychological barriers. Barriers may include the inaccessibility of facilities and the lack of staff trained in working with people with disabilities.

A multidisciplinary approach to promoting physical activity brings about traditional partnerships, such as that of education and health care, with nontraditional partnerships representing, for example, transportation, urban planning, recreation, and environmental health. Data sources that are representative of the entire Nation are needed to monitor key characteristics of the environment, such as the availability of parks and trails, the usage of these spaces, and policies that promote physical activity at worksites, in communities, and in schools.

PREPAREDNESS

Preparedness involves Government agencies, nongovernmental organizations, the private sector, communities, and individuals working together to improve the Nation's ability to prevent, prepare for, respond to, and recover from a major health incident. The objectives for preparedness are based on a set of national priorities articulated in the National Health Security Strategy of the United States of America (NHSS). The overarching goals of NHSS are to build community resilience and to strengthen and sustain health and emergency response systems.

To reach these goals, NHSS identifies the following objectives for urgent, focused attention:

- Foster informed, empowered individuals and communities.
- Develop and maintain the workforce needed for national health security.
- Ensure situational awareness.
- Foster integrated, scalable health care delivery systems.
- Ensure timely and effective communications.
- Promote an effective countermeasure enterprise.
- Ensure prevention or mitigation of environmental and other emerging threats to health.
- Incorporate postincident health recovery into planning and response.
- Work with cross-border and global partners to enhance national, continental, and global health security.
- Ensure that all systems that support national health security are based on the best available science, evaluation, and quality improvement.

The United States, like all countries, faces many threats with the potential for large-scale health consequences, including disease outbreaks, natural disasters, and terrorist attacks. The public health, health care, and emergency response systems must be prepared to mitigate the morbidity and mortality associated with these threats. Securing the Nation's health is a formidable task, and it is a shared responsibility for virtually all parts of society.

Many factors determine a community's level of preparedness and its ability to recover after an emergency. These factors include:

- The general health of a population
- Individual behaviors, lifestyles, and social interconnectedness
- Individual community members planning and preparing for an emergency
- Economic and social conditions
- Having broad and prepared health services
- Access to health services

Over the decade, more communities will focus on improving their ability to withstand, recover, and learn from an emergency. To become resilient communities, they will need to:

- Account for and address their vulnerabilities.

- Develop capabilities that aid the community in preventing, withstanding, and mitigating the stress of a health incident.
- Recover in a way that moves the community to a state of self-sufficiency and at least the same level of health and social functioning following adversity as before it, if not better.
- Use knowledge gained from 1 incident to strengthen the community's ability to withstand the next.

Additional research and experiences will likely reinforce the importance of the following factors that contribute to a community's preparedness and resilience:

- Informed and empowered communities
- Preincident planning that engages citizens and at-risk individuals
- Social interconnectedness
- Robust and prepared infrastructures for health services
- Availability of nongovernmental sources of assistance during and after an incident

PUBLIC HEALTH INFRASTRUCTURE

Public health infrastructure is fundamental to the provision and execution of public health services at all levels. A strong infrastructure provides the capacity to prepare for and respond to both acute (emergency) and chronic (ongoing) threats to the Nation's health. Infrastructure is the foundation for planning, delivering, and evaluating public health.

Why Is Public Health Infrastructure Important?

Public health infrastructure includes three key components that enable a public health organization at the Federal, Tribal, State, or local level to deliver public health services. These components are:

- A capable and qualified workforce
- Up-to-date data and information systems
- Public health agencies capable of assessing and responding to public health needs

These components are necessary to fulfill the following 10 Essential Public Health Services:

Monitor health status to identify and solve community health problems.

Diagnose and investigate health problems and health hazards in the community.

Inform, educate, and empower people about health issues.

Mobilize community partnerships and action to identify and solve health problems.

Develop policies and plans that support individual and community health efforts.

Enforce laws and regulations that protect health and ensure safety.

Link people to needed personal health services and assure the provision of health care when otherwise unavailable.

Ensure competent public and personal health care workforces.

Evaluate effectiveness, accessibility, and quality of personal and population-based health services.

Research for new insights and innovative solutions to health problems.

Public Health Infrastructure allows for and supports key goals of Healthy People, including the:

- Improvement of health
- Creation of environments that promote good health
- Promotion of healthy development and behaviors

Public health infrastructure, along with the 10 essential functions of public health, influences—and is influenced by—a number of factors, including the social and political environment. As such, public health infrastructure provides a useful framework for addressing the social determinants of health.

Increasing attention to public health infrastructure has led to the identification of a number of emerging issues. As minority populations in the United States increase, the country will need a more diverse public health workforce. Hispanics, American Indians and Alaska Natives, and African Americans are underrepresented in the public health workforce.

In an effort to standardize services and improve performance, public health agencies are moving toward a voluntary national accreditation program. This program will highlight agencies' commitment to service and quality and provide a standard toward which all public health agencies can work.

Expanding the evidence base for community interventions and for the effective organization, administration, and financing of public health services is critical to the future development of public health infrastructure. The emerging field of public health systems and services research is playing an important role in the development of this evidence base; its role should be supported and expanded over the decade, with a strong focus on translating research into practice.

Novel policies are being developed to address legal and political challenges resulting from new and re-emerging infectious diseases and increasing levels of chronic disease. New centers devoted to the study of public health law are adding to the body of knowledge in this critical area.

RESPIRATORY DISEASES

Asthma and chronic obstructive pulmonary disease (COPD) are significant public health burdens. Specific methods of detection, intervention, and treatment exist that may reduce this burden and promote health.

Asthma is a chronic inflammatory disorder of the airways characterized by episodes of reversible breathing problems due to airway narrowing and obstruction. These episodes can range in severity from mild to life threatening. Symptoms of asthma include wheezing, coughing, chest tightness, and shortness of breath. Daily preventive treatment can prevent symptoms and attacks and enable individuals who have asthma to lead active lives.

COPD is a preventable and treatable disease characterized by airflow limitation that is not fully reversible. The airflow limitation is usually progressive and associated with an abnormal inflammatory response of the lung to noxious particles or gases (typically from exposure to cigarette smoke). Treatment can lessen symptoms and improve quality of life for those with COPD.

Several additional respiratory conditions and respiratory hazards tuberculosis, lung cancer, acquired immunodeficiency syndrome (AIDS), pneumonia, occupational lung disease, and smoking.

Currently in the United States, more than 23 million people have asthma. Approximately 13.6 million adults have been diagnosed with COPD, and an approximately equal number have not yet been diagnosed. The burden of respiratory diseases affects individuals and their families, schools, workplaces, neighborhoods, cities, and states. Because of the cost to the health care system, the burden of respiratory diseases also falls on society; it is paid for with higher health insurance rates, lost productivity, and tax dollars. Annual health care expenditures for asthma alone are estimated at $20.7 billion.

The prevalence of asthma has increased since 1980. However, deaths from asthma have decreased since the mid-1990s. The causes of asthma are an active area of research and involve both genetic and environmental factors. Risk factors for asthma currently being investigated include:

- Having a parent with asthma
- Sensitization to irritants and allergens
- Respiratory infections in childhood
- Overweight

Asthma affects people of every race, sex, and age. However, significant disparities in asthma morbidity and mortality exist, in particular for low-income and minority populations. Populations with higher rates of asthma include:

- Children
- Women (among adults) and boys (among children)
- African Americans
- Puerto Ricans
- People living in the Northeast United States
- People living below the Federal poverty level
- Employees with certain exposures in the workplace

While there is not a cure for asthma yet, there are diagnoses and treatment guidelines that are aimed at ensuring that all people with asthma live full and active lives.

COPD is the fourth leading cause of death in the United States. In 2006, approximately 120,000 individuals died from COPD, a number very close to that reported for lung cancer deaths (approximately 158,600) in the same year. In nearly 8 out of 10 cases, COPD is caused by exposure to cigarette smoke. In addition, other environmental exposures (such as those in the workplace) may cause COPD.

Genetic factors strongly influence the development of the disease. For example, not all smokers develop COPD. Quitting smoking may slow the progression of the disease. Women and men are affected equally, yet more women than men have died of COPD since 2000.

It should be recognized that there are other important respiratory diseases. Examples include idiopathic pulmonary fibrosis, sarcoidosis, respiratory distress syndromes, and upper airway conditions, such as rhinitis and chronic sinusitis. In some cases, effective preventive interventions do not exist. In others, nationally representative trend data for disease prevalence and/or incidence, causative exposures, and other preventable risk factors are not available for tracking of measurable goals. It is hoped that, as preventive interventions and surveillance for respiratory hazards and diseases continue to improve, measurable goals for at least some of these additional respiratory hazards and diseases will be available.

Other emerging issues in the Respiratory Diseases topic area include:

- Assessing the impact of climate change (temperature extremes, the increased geographic span of allergens, and air quality) on asthma causation and exacerbations.
- Increasing importance of indoor air quality as a cause of work-related respiratory symptoms and asthma in a service economy.
- Increasing use of nanotechnology and resulting exposures to engineered nanoparticles.
- Increasing exposures to respiratory hazards such as isocyanates used in "green" building materials.
- Applying knowledge about gene-environment interactions and epigenetics to respiratory disease prevention.
- Using knowledge about primary causes of asthma (determination of distinct asthma phenotypes) in developing effective prevention strategies, such as weight control and allergen avoidance.
- Developing novel treatments to alter the progression of disease severity and, ultimately, to prevent asthma onset.
- Using personalized medicine (tailoring treatment to a patient's specific phenotype, genetics, and history).
- Identifying new respiratory hazards, as has been done during the last decade for diacetyl and other butter-flavoring chemicals; nylon, rayon, and polypropylene flock; and World Trade Center dust.
- Improving COPD awareness and clinical case-finding in the population at large, and in the health care delivery system at the State and local levels.
- Establishing a surveillance system for COPD.

SEXUALLY TRANSMITTED DISEASES (STDS)

STDs refer to more than 25 infectious organisms that are transmitted primarily through sexual activity. STD prevention is an essential primary care strategy for improving reproductive health.

Despite their burdens, costs, and complications, and the fact that they are largely preventable, STDs remain a significant public health problem in the United States. This problem is largely unrecognized by the public, policymakers, and health care professionals. STDs cause many harmful, often irreversible, and costly clinical complications, such as:

- Reproductive health problems
- Fetal and perinatal health problems
- Cancer
- Facilitation of the sexual transmission of HIV infection

The Centers for Disease Control and Prevention (CDC) estimates that there are approximately 19 million new STD infections each year—almost half of them among young people ages 15 to 24. The cost of STDs to the U.S. health care system is estimated to be as much as $15.9 billion annually. Because many cases of STDs go undiagnosed—and some common viral infections, such as human papillomavirus (HPV) and genital herpes, are not reported to CDC at all—the reported cases of chlamydia, gonorrhea, and syphilis represent only a fraction of the true burden of STDs in the United States.

Untreated STDs can lead to serious long-term health consequences, especially for adolescent girls and young women. CDC estimates that undiagnosed and untreated STDs cause at least 24,000 women in the United States each year to become infertile.

Several factors contribute to the spread of STDs. STDs are acquired during unprotected sex with an infected partner. Biological factors that affect the spread of STDs include:

- Asymptomatic nature of STDs. The majority of STDs either do not produce any symptoms or signs, or they produce symptoms so mild that they are unnoticed; consequently, many infected persons do not know that they need medical care.
- Gender disparities. Women suffer more frequent and more serious STD complications than men do. Among the most serious STD complications are pelvic inflammatory disease, ectopic pregnancy (pregnancy outside of the uterus), infertility, and chronic pelvic pain.

- Age disparities. Compared to older adults, sexually active adolescents ages 15 to 19 and young adults ages 20 to 24 are at higher risk for getting STDs.
- Lag time between infection and complications. Often, a long interval, sometimes years, occurs between acquiring an STD and recognizing a clinically significant health problem.

The spread of STDs is directly affected by social, economic, and behavioral factors. Such factors may cause serious obstacles to STD prevention due to their influence on social and sexual networks, access to and provision of care, willingness to seek care, and social norms regarding sex and sexuality. Among certain vulnerable populations, historical experience with segregation and discrimination exacerbates the influence of these factors. Social, economic, and behavioral factors that affect the spread of STDs include:

- Racial and ethnic disparities. Certain racial and ethnic groups (mainly African American, Hispanic, and American Indian/Alaska Native populations) have high rates of STDs, compared with rates for whites. Race and ethnicity in the United States are correlated with other determinants of health status, such as poverty, limited access to health care, fewer attempts to get medical treatment, and living in communities with high rates of STDs.
- Poverty and marginalization. STDs disproportionately affect disenfranchised people and people in social networks where high-risk sexual behavior is common, and either access to care or health-seeking behavior is compromised.
- Access to health care. Access to high-quality health care is essential for early detection, treatment, and behavior-change counseling for STDs. Groups with the highest rates of STDs are often the same groups for whom access to or use of health services is most limited.
- Substance abuse. Many studies document the association of substance abuse with STDs. The introduction of new illicit substances into communities often can alter sexual behavior drastically in high-risk sexual networks, leading to the epidemic spread of STDs.
- Sexuality and secrecy. Perhaps the most important social factors contributing to the spread of STDs in the United States are the stigma associated with STDs and the general discomfort of discussing intimate aspects of life, especially those related to sex. These social factors separate the United States from industrialized countries with low rates of STDs.

- Sexual networks. Sexual networks refer to groups of people who can be considered "linked" by sequential or concurrent sexual partners. A person may have only one sex partner, but if that partner is a member of a risky sexual network, then the person is at higher risk for STDs than a similar individual from a nonrisky network.

There are several emerging issues in STD prevention:

- Each State needs to address system-level barriers to the implementation of expedited partner therapy for the treatment of chlamydia and gonorrheal infections.
- Enhanced data collection on demographic and behavioral variables, such as the sex of an infected person's sex partner(s), is essential to understanding the epidemiology of STDs and to guiding prevention efforts.
- Innovative communication strategies are critical for addressing issues of disparities, facilitating HPV vaccine uptake, and normalizing perceptions of sexual health and STD prevention, particularly as they help reduce health disparities.
- It is necessary to coordinate STD prevention efforts with the health care delivery system to leverage new developments provided by health reform legislation.

SLEEP HEALTH

Poor sleep health is a common problem with 25 percent of U.S. adults reporting insufficient sleep or rest at least 15 out of every 30 days. The public health burden of chronic sleep loss and sleep disorders, coupled with low awareness of poor sleep health among the general population, health care professionals, and policymakers, necessitates a well-coordinated strategy to improve sleep-related health.

Sleep, like nutrition and physical activity, is a critical determinant of health and well-being. Sleep is a basic requirement for infant, child, and adolescent health and development. Sleep loss and untreated sleep disorders influence basic patterns of behavior that negatively affect family health and interpersonal relationships. Fatigue and sleepiness can reduce productivity and increase the chance for mishaps such as medical errors and motor vehicle or industrial accidents. Adequate sleep is necessary to:

- Fight off infection
- Support the metabolism of sugar to prevent diabetes
- Perform well in school
- Work effectively and safely

Sleep timing and duration affect a number of endocrine, metabolic, and neurological functions that are critical to the maintenance of individual health. If left untreated, sleep disorders and chronic short sleep are associated with an increased risk of:

- Heart disease
- High blood pressure
- Obesity
- Diabetes
- All-cause mortality

Sleep health is a particular concern for individuals with chronic disabilities and disorders such as arthritis, kidney disease, pain, human immunodeficiency virus (HIV), epilepsy, Parkinson's disease, and depression. Among older adults, the cognitive and medical consequences of untreated sleep disorders decrease health-related quality of life, contribute to functional limitations and loss of independence, and are associated with an increased risk of death from any cause.

The odds of being a short sleeper (defined as someone who sleeps less than 6 hours a night) in the United States have increased significantly over the past 30 years. Competition between sleep schedules, employment, and lifestyle is a recent trend. Intermittent sleep disturbances due to lifestyle choices are associated with temporary fatigue, disorientation, and decreased alertness.

Sleep-disordered breathing (SDB), which includes sleep apnea, is another serious threat to health. SDB is characterized by intermittent airway obstruction or pauses in breathing. People with untreated SDB have 2 to 4 times the risk of heart attack and stroke. Obesity is a significant risk factor for SDB, and weight loss is associated with a decrease in SDB severity.

SDB in Children:

African American children are at least twice as likely to develop SDB than children of European descent. The risk of SDB during childhood is associated with low socioeconomic status independent of obesity and other risk factors. Left untreated, SDB in children is associated with difficulties in school, metabolic disorders, and future heart disease risk.

SDB in Older Adults:

SDB may affect 20 to 40 percent of older adults and, if left untreated, is associated with a 2- to 3-fold increased risk of stroke and mortality.

Sleep health education and promotion strategies are needed to address disparities in sleep health across age, race, education, and socioeconomic groups. Health education and promotion programs can increase awareness of common sleep disorders, such as insomnia, restless leg syndrome, and SDB. Sleep health education programs in workplaces can promote better work schedule patterns and motivate managers and workers to adopt strategies that reduce risks to health and safety. Without sleep health education, individuals often prioritize other activities over sleep and accept constant sleepiness and sleep disruption as inevitable.

Progress in the following areas will yield more information on sleep health over the coming decade:

- Further evolution of biomedical sleep research
- Quantification of health risks associated with untreated SDB across the lifespan
- Findings from the first U.S.-based phase III SDB treatment trials in children and adults

SOCIAL DETERMINANTS OF HEALTH

Health starts in our homes, schools, workplaces, neighborhoods, and communities. We know that taking care of ourselves by eating well and staying active, not smoking, getting the recommended immunizations and screening tests, and seeing a doctor when we are sick all influence our health. Our health is also determined in part by access to social and economic opportunities; the resources and supports available in our homes, neighborhoods, and communities; the quality of our schooling; the safety of our workplaces; the cleanliness of our water, food, and air; and the nature of our social interactions and relationships. The conditions in which we live explain in part why some Americans are healthier than others and why Americans more generally are not as healthy as they could be.

The importance of addressing the social determinants of health is shared by the World Health Organization, whose Commission on Social Determinants of Health in 2008 published the report, Closing the gap in a generation: Health equity through action on the social determinants of health. The emphasis is also shared by other U.S. health initiatives such as the National Partnership for Action to End Health Disparities and the National Prevention and Health Promotion Strategy.

All Americans deserve an equal opportunity to make the choices that lead to good health. But to ensure that all Americans have that opportunity, advances are needed not only in health care but also in fields such as education, childcare, housing, business, law, media, community planning, transportation, and agriculture. Making these advances involves working together to:

- Explore how programs, practices, and policies in these areas affect the health of individuals, families, and communities.
- Establish common goals, complementary roles, and ongoing constructive relationships between the health sector and these areas.
- Maximize opportunities for collaboration among Federal-, state-, and local-level partners related to social determinants of health.

Social determinants of health are conditions in the environments in which people are born, live, learn, work, play, worship, and age that affect a wide range of health, functioning, and quality-of-life outcomes and risks. Conditions (e.g., social, economic, and physical) in these various environments and settings (e.g., school, church, workplace, and neighborhood) have been referred to as "place." In addition to the more material attributes of "place," the patterns of social engagement and sense of security and well-being are also affected by where people live. Resources that enhance quality of life can have a significant influence on population health outcomes. Examples of these resources include safe and affordable housing, access to education, public safety, availability of healthy foods, local emergency/health services, and environments free of life-threatening toxins.

Understanding the relationship between how population groups experience "place" and the impact of "place" on health is fundamental to the social determinants of health—including both social and physical determinants. Examples of social determinants include:

- Availability of resources to meet daily needs (e.g., safe housing and local food markets)
- Access to educational, economic, and job opportunities
- Access to health care services
- Quality of education and job training
- Availability of community-based resources in support of community living and opportunities for recreational and leisure-time activities

- Transportation options
- Public safety
- Social support
- Social norms and attitudes (e.g., discrimination, racism, and distrust of government)
- Exposure to crime, violence, and social disorder (e.g., presence of trash and lack of cooperation in a community)
- Socioeconomic conditions (e.g., concentrated poverty and the stressful conditions that accompany it)
- Residential segregation
- Language/Literacy
- Access to mass media and emerging technologies (e.g., cell phones, the Internet, and social media)
- Culture

Examples of physical determinants include:

- Natural environment, such as green space (e.g., trees and grass) or weather (e.g., climate change)
- Built environment, such as buildings, sidewalks, bike lanes, and roads
- Worksites, schools, and recreational settings
- Housing and community design
- Exposure to toxic substances and other physical hazards
- Physical barriers, especially for people with disabilities
- Aesthetic elements (e.g., good lighting, trees, and benches)

By working to establish policies that positively influence social and economic conditions and those that support changes in individual behavior, we can improve health for large numbers of people in ways that can be sustained over time. Improving the conditions in which we live, learn, work, and play and the quality of our relationships will create a healthier population, society, and workforce.

- Economic Stability
- Education
- Social and Community Context
- Health and Health Care
- Neighborhood and Built Environment

Each of these five determinant areas reflects a number of critical components/key issues that make up the underlying factors in the arena of SDOH.

- Economic Stability
- Poverty

- Employment
- Food Security
- Housing Stability
- Education
- High School Graduation
- Enrollment in Higher Education
- Language and Literacy
- Early Childhood Education and Development
- Social and Community Context
- Social Cohesion
- Civic Participation
- Perceptions of Discrimination and Equity
- Incarceration/Institutionalization
- Health and Health Care
- Access to Health Care
- Access to Primary Care
- Health Literacy
- Neighborhood and Built Environment
- Access to Healthy Foods
- Quality of Housing
- Crime and Violence
- Environmental Conditions

A number of tools and strategies are emerging to address the social determinants of health, including:

- Use of Health Impact Assessments to review needed, proposed, and existing social policies for their likely impact on health
- Application of a "health in all policies" strategy, which introduces improved health for all and the closing of health gaps as goals to be shared across all areas of government

SUBSTANCE ABUSE

An estimated 22 million Americans struggle with a drug or alcohol problem. Almost 95 percent of people with substance use problems are considered unaware of their problem. Of those who recognize their problem, 273,000 have made an unsuccessful effort to obtain treatment. These estimates highlight the importance of increasing prevention efforts and improving access to treatment for substance abuse and co-occurring disorders.

Substance abuse has a major impact on individuals, families, and communities. The effects of substance abuse are cumulative, significantly contributing to costly social, physical, mental, and public health problems. These problems include:

- Teenage pregnancy
- Human immunodeficiency virus/acquired immunodeficiency syndrome (HIV/AIDS)
- Other sexually transmitted diseases (STDs)
- Domestic violence
- Child abuse
- Motor vehicle crashes
- Physical fights
- Crime
- Homicide
- Suicide

Substance abuse refers to a set of related conditions associated with the consumption of mind- and behavior-altering substances that have negative behavioral and health outcomes. Social attitudes and political and legal responses to the consumption of alcohol and illicit drugs make substance abuse one of the most complex public health issues. In addition to the considerable health implications, substance abuse has been a flash-point in the criminal justice system and a major focal point in discussions about social values: people argue over whether substance abuse is a disease with genetic and biological foundations or a matter of personal choice.

Advances in research have led to the development of evidence-based strategies to effectively address substance abuse.

Improvements in brain-imaging technologies and the development of medications that assist in treatment have gradually shifted the research community's perspective on substance abuse. There is now a deeper understanding of substance abuse as a disorder that develops in adolescence and, for some individuals, will develop into a chronic illness that will require lifelong monitoring and care.

Improved evaluation of community-level prevention has enhanced researchers' understanding of environmental and social factors that contribute to the initiation and abuse of alcohol and illicit drugs, leading to a more sophisticated understanding of how to implement evidence-based strategies in specific social and cultural settings.

A stronger emphasis on evaluation has expanded evidence-based practices for drug and alcohol treatment. Improvements have focused on the development of better clinical interventions through research and increasing the skills and qualifications of treatment providers.

In recent years, the impact of substance and alcohol abuse has been notable across several areas, including the following:

Adolescent abuse of prescription drugs has continued to rise over the past 5 years. The 2007 MTF survey found high rates of nonmedical use of the prescription pain relievers Vicodin and OxyContin. It is believed that 2 factors have led to the increase in abuse. First, the availability of prescription drugs is increasing from many sources, including the family medicine cabinet, the Internet, and doctors. Second, many adolescents believe that prescription drugs are safer to take than street drugs.

Military operations in Iraq and Afghanistan have placed a great strain on military personnel and their families. This strain can lead to family disintegration, mental health disorders, and even suicide. Data from the Substance Abuse and Mental Health Services Administration (SAMSHA) National Survey on Drug Use and Health indicate that 7.1 percent of veterans (an estimated 1.8 million people) had a substance use disorder in the past year.

In addition, as the Federal Government begins to implement health reform legislation, it will focus attention on providing services for individuals with mental illness and substance use disorders, including new opportunities for access to and coverage of treatment and prevention services.

TOBACCO USE

Scientific knowledge about the health effects of tobacco use has increased greatly since the first Surgeon General's report on tobacco was released in 1964. Tobacco use causes:
- Cancer
- Heart disease

- Lung diseases (including emphysema, bronchitis, and chronic airway obstruction)
- Premature birth, low birth weight, stillbirth, and infant death

There is no risk-free level of exposure to secondhand smoke. Secondhand smoke causes heart disease and lung cancer in adults and a number of health problems in infants and children, including:

- Severe asthma attacks
- Respiratory infections
- Ear infections
- Sudden infant death syndrome (SIDS)

Smokeless tobacco causes a number of serious oral health problems, including cancer of the mouth and gums, periodontitis, and tooth loss. Cigar use causes cancer of the larynx, mouth, esophagus, and lung.

Tobacco use is the single most preventable cause of death and disease in the United States. Each year, approximately 443,000 Americans die from tobacco-related illnesses. For every person who dies from tobacco use, 20 more people suffer with at least 1 serious tobacco-related illness. In addition, tobacco use costs the U.S. $193 billion annually in direct medical expenses and lost productivity.

The goal is to reduce tobacco use to the point that it is no longer a public health problem for the Nation. Research has identified a number of effective strategies that will contribute to ending tobacco use. Based on more than 45 years of evidence, it is clear that the toll tobacco use takes on families and communities can be significantly reduced by:

- Fully funding tobacco control programs.
- Increasing the price of tobacco products.
- Enacting comprehensive smoke-free policies.
- Controlling access to tobacco products.
- Reducing tobacco advertising and promotion.
- Implementing anti-tobacco media campaigns.
- Encouraging and assisting tobacco users to quit.

The strategy to reduce tobacco use is organized into 3 key areas:

Tobacco Use Prevalence: Implementing policies to reduce tobacco use and initiation among youth and adults.

Health System Changes: Adopting policies and strategies to increase access, affordability, and use of smoking cessation services and treatments.

Social and Environmental Changes: Establishing policies to reduce exposure to secondhand smoke, increase the cost of tobacco, restrict tobacco advertising, and reduce illegal sales to minors.

Preventing tobacco use and helping tobacco users quit can improve the health and quality of life for Americans of all ages. People who stop smoking greatly reduce their risk of disease and premature death. Benefits are greater for people who stop at earlier ages, but quitting tobacco use is beneficial at any age.

Many factors influence tobacco use, disease, and mortality. Risk factors include race/ethnicity, age, education, and socioeconomic status. Significant disparities in tobacco use exist geographically; such disparities typically result from differences among states in smoke-free protections, tobacco prices, and program funding for tobacco prevention.

In the last five years, 25 states and the District of Columbia (DC) have enacted comprehensive smoke-free laws eliminating smoking in workplaces, restaurants, and bars, and 14 States and DC have cigarette excise tax rates of at least $2 per pack. Over the coming decade, more States are poised to strengthen smoke-free laws and increase the price of tobacco, further reducing tobacco use and initiation throughout the Nation.

VISION

Vision is an essential part of everyday life, influencing how Americans of all ages learn, communicate, work, play, and interact with the world. Yet millions of Americans live with visual impairment, and many more remain at risk for eye disease and preventable eye injury.

Strategies to preserve sight and prevent blindness must address screening and examinations for children and adults, early detection and timely treatment of eye diseases and conditions, injury prevention, and the use of vision rehabilitation services.

The eyes are an important, but often overlooked, part of overall health. Despite the preventable nature of some vision impairments, many people do not receive recommended screenings and exams. A visit to an eye care professional for a comprehensive dilated eye exam can help to detect common vision problems and eye diseases, including:

- Diabetic retinopathy
- Glaucoma
- Cataract
- Age-related macular degeneration (AMD)

These common vision problems often have no early warning signs. If a problem is detected, an eye care professional can prescribe corrective eyewear, medicine, or surgery to minimize vision loss and help a person see his or her best. Healthy vision can help keep people safe when behind the wheel, participating in sports, or working with power tools in the yard or around the home. It can also help to ensure a healthy and active lifestyle well into a person's later years. Educating and engaging families, communities, and the Nation is critical to ensuring that people have the information, resources, and tools needed for good eye health. Resources and tools include:

- Eye health care
- Vision correction
- Emerging treatments
- Vision rehabilitation services and adaptive devices that enable people to make the most of their remaining vision and maintain an independent lifestyle

The need to promote and protect healthy vision continues through the entire lifespan and applies to all ethnic and racial groups. Research indicates that several diseases and eye disorders are more prevalent in certain racial and ethnic minority communities and disproportionately affect minority populations more than whites.

In 2005, the National Eye Institute (NEI) conducted a series of focus groups on factors that influence the receipt of preventive eye care. Participants indicated that the cost of services is prohibitive, particularly when it comes to receiving follow-up care.

With the aging of the population, the number of Americans with major eye diseases is increasing, and vision loss is becoming a major public health concern. By the year 2020, the number of people who are blind or have low vision is projected to reach 5.5 million.

Eye injuries are also a major eye health concern in the United States. Each day, more than 2,000 American workers receive some form of medical treatment due to eye injuries that happen at work. Nearly half of all eye injuries occur at home, and more than 1 in 4 occur during sporting and recreational activities, or on streets and highways.

Researchers are capitalizing on the remarkable progress made by the Human Genome Project and the Genome-Wide Association Studies. Datasets for AMD and a twin study of risk factors for glaucoma and myopia have been added to the public domain (known as dBGap). New studies are also working to identify the relationships of environmental exposures to gene-trait associations in common, complex diseases.

Gene transfer therapy in patients with Leber congenital amaurosis—a severe, early-onset retinal disease—indicates that the treatment is safe, with evidence of lasting visual improvement. These findings could help usher gene-based therapies for other retinal diseases, such as retinitis pigmentosa and macular degeneration, into clinical trials.

Investigators are conducting several comparative effectiveness clinical trials to improve ophthalmic care.

- Laser treatment is a standard of care for diabetic eye disease, where abnormal blood vessel growth damages the retina. However, recent evidence suggests that treatment with various drugs may deliver a better outcome.
- Researchers aim to understand the complex genetic and biological factors that cause glaucoma and to develop treatments that protect optic nerves from the damage that leads to vision loss.

Rehabilitation research is improving the quality of life of people with visual impairments by helping them maximize the use of remaining vision and by devising improved aids and strategies to assist those without useful vision.

2

Heart Disease, Heart Failure, and Stroke

HEART DISEASE

Heart disease is the leading cause of death in America today and costs the nation $300 billion each year. Major factors in the development of heart disease include high blood pressure, high cholesterol and smoking. Some medical conditions and lifestyle habits can also influence heart disease, including diabetes, obesity, stagnant lifestyle, incorrect diet choices and alcoholism. Many heart disease prevention campaigns have been launched over the years, and most recently, the Department of Health and Human Services, along with the American Heart Association, have initiated Million Hearts, which strives to prevent 1 million strokes and heart attacks by 2017.

For both men and women, heart disease kills the largest number of Americans per year. According to the American Heart Association, heart disease, which causes heart attacks and strokes, kills more people than all forms of cancer combined. Quit smoking and eat a diet low in fat and sodium to cut your risk.

America's Heart Disease Burden

About 610,000 people die of heart disease in the United States every year–that's 1 in every 4 deaths.

Heart disease is the leading cause of death for both men and women. Coronary heart disease is the most common type of heart disease, killing nearly 380,000 people annually.

Every year about 735,000 Americans have a heart attack. Of these, 525,000 are a first heart attack and 210,000 happen in people who have already had a heart attack.

Coronary heart disease alone costs the United States $108.9 billion each year. This total includes the cost of health care services, medications, and lost productivity.

Deaths Vary by Ethnicity

Heart disease is the leading cause of death for people of most ethnicities in the United States, including African Americans, Hispanics, and whites. For American Indians or Alaska Natives and Asians or Pacific Islanders, heart disease is second only to cancer.

Men and Heart Disease

Heart disease is the leading cause of death for men of most racial/ethnic groups in the United States, including African Americans, American Indians or Alaska Natives, Hispanics, and whites. For Asian American or Pacific Islander men, heart disease is second only to cancer.

About 8.5% of all white men, 7.9% of black men, and 6.3% of Mexican American men have coronary heart disease.

Half of the men who die suddenly of coronary heart disease have no previous symptoms. Even if you have no symptoms, you may still be at risk for heart disease.

Between 70% and 89% of sudden cardiac events occur in men.

Women and Heart Disease

Heart disease is the leading cause of death for women in the United States, killing around 290,000 women a year.

Although heart disease is sometimes thought of as a "man's disease," around the same number of women and men die each year of heart disease in the United States. Despite increases in awareness over the past decade, only 54% of women recognize that heart disease is their number 1 killer.

Heart disease is the leading cause of death for African American and white women in the United States. Among Hispanic women, heart disease and cancer cause roughly the same number of deaths each year. For American Indian or Alaska Native and Asian or Pacific Islander women, heart disease is second only to cancer.

About 5.8% of all white women, 7.6% of black women, and 5.6% of Mexican American women have coronary heart disease.

Almost two-thirds (64%) of women who die suddenly of coronary heart disease have no previous symptoms. Even if you have no symptoms, you may still be at risk for heart disease.

Symptoms

While some women have no symptoms, others experience angina (dull, heavy to sharp chest pain or discomfort), pain in the neck/jaw/throat or pain in the upper abdomen or back. These may occur during rest, begin during physical activity, or be triggered by mental stress.

Women are more likely to describe chest pain that is sharp, burning and more frequently have pain in the neck, jaw, throat, abdomen or back.

Sometimes heart disease may be silent and not diagnosed until a woman experiences signs or symptoms of a heart attack, heart failure, an arrhythmia, or stroke.

These symptoms may include

Heart Attack: Chest pain or discomfort, upper back pain, indigestion, heartburn, nausea/vomiting, extreme fatigue, upper body discomfort, and shortness of breath.

Arrhythmia: Fluttering feelings in the chest (palpitations).

Heart Failure: Shortness of breath, fatigue, swelling of the feet/ankles/legs/abdomen.

Stroke: Sudden weakness, paralysis (inability to move) or numbness of the face/arms/legs, especially on one side of the body. Other symptoms may include: confusion, trouble speaking or understanding speech, difficulty seeing in one or both eyes, shortness of breath, dizziness, loss of balance or coordination, loss of consciousness, or sudden and severe headache.

Early Action is Key

To reduce your chances of getting heart disease it's important to:

- Know your blood pressure. Having uncontrolled blood pressure can result in heart disease. High blood pressure has no symptoms so it's important to have your blood pressure checked regularly.
- Talk to your healthcare provider about whether you should be tested for diabetes. Having uncontrolled diabetes raises your chances of heart disease.
- Quit smoking.
- Discuss checking your cholesterol and triglycerides with your healthcare provider.
- Make healthy food choices. Being overweight and obese raises your risk of heart disease.
- Limit alcohol intake to one drink a day.
- Lower your stress level and find healthy ways to cope with stress.

Knowing the warning signs and symptoms of a heart attack is key to preventing death, but many people don't know the signs.

In a 2005 survey, most respondents—92%—recognized chest pain as a symptom of a heart attack. Only 27% were aware of all major symptoms and knew to call 9-1-1 when someone was having a heart attack.

About 47% of sudden cardiac deaths occur outside a hospital. This suggests that many people with heart disease don't act on early warning signs.

Heart attacks have several major warning signs and symptoms:

- Chest pain or discomfort.
- Upper body pain or discomfort in the arms, back, neck, jaw, or upper stomach.
- Shortness of breath.
- Nausea, lightheadedness, or cold sweats.

High blood pressure, high LDL cholesterol, and smoking are key risk factors for heart disease. About half of Americans (49%) have at least one of these three risk factors.

Several other medical conditions and lifestyle choices can also put people at a higher risk for heart disease, including:

- Diabetes
- Overweight and obesity
- Poor diet
- Physical inactivity

- Excessive alcohol use

Protect Your Heart

Lowering your blood pressure and cholesterol will reduce your risk of dying of heart disease. Here are some tips to protect your heart:
- Follow your doctor's instructions and stay on your medications.
- Eat a healthy diet that is low in salt; low in total fat, saturated fat, and cholesterol; and rich in fresh fruits and vegetables.
- Take a brisk 10-minute walk, 3 times a day, 5 days a week.
- Don't smoke. If you smoke, quit as soon as possible

For more tips on quitting smoking visit www.cdc.gov/tobacco and www.smokefree.gov.

HEART FAILURE

Heart failure is a condition in which the heart can't pump enough blood to meet the body's needs. In some cases, the heart can't fill with enough blood. In other cases, the heart can't pump blood to the rest of the body with enough force. Some people have both problems.

The term "heart failure" doesn't mean that your heart has stopped or is about to stop working. However, heart failure is a serious condition that requires medical care.

Heart failure develops over time as the heart's pumping action grows weaker. The condition can affect the right side of the heart only, or it can affect both sides of the heart. Most cases involve both sides of the heart. Right-side heart failure occurs if the heart can't pump enough blood to the lungs to pick up oxygen. Left-side heart failure occurs if the heart can't pump enough oxygen-rich blood to the rest of the body.

Right-side heart failure may cause fluid to build up in the feet, ankles, legs, liver, abdomen, and the veins in the neck. Right-side and left-side heart failure also may cause shortness of breath and fatigue (tiredness).

Heart failure is a very common condition. About 5.1 million people in the United States have heart failure. Both children and adults can have the condition, although the symptoms and treatments differ.

Currently, heart failure has no cure. However, treatments—such as medicines and lifestyle changes—can help people who have the condition live longer and more active lives. Researchers continue to study new ways to treat heart failure and its complications.

Causes of Heart Failure

The leading causes of heart failure are diseases that damage the heart. Examples include coronary heart disease (CHD), high blood pressure, and diabetes.

Coronary Heart Disease (CHD)

CHD is a condition in which a waxy substance called plaque builds up inside the coronary arteries. These arteries supply oxygen-rich blood to your heart muscle. Plaque narrows the arteries and reduces blood flow to your heart muscle. The buildup of plaque also makes it more likely that blood clots will form in your arteries. Blood clots can partially or completely block blood flow.

CHD can lead to chest pain or discomfort called angina, a heart attack, heart damage, or even death.

High Blood Pressure

Blood pressure is the force of blood pushing against the walls of the arteries. If this pressure rises and stays high over time, it can weaken your heart and lead to plaque buildup. Blood pressure is considered high if it stays at or above 140/90 mmHg over time. (The mmHg is millimeters of mercury—the units used to measure blood pressure.) If you have diabetes or chronic kidney disease, high blood pressure is defined as 130/80 mmHg or higher.

Diabetes

Diabetes is a disease in which the body's blood glucose (sugar) level is too high. The body normally breaks down food into glucose and then carries it to cells throughout the body. The cells use a hormone called insulin to turn the glucose into energy. In diabetes, the body doesn't make enough insulin or doesn't use its insulin properly. Over time, high blood sugar levels can damage and weaken the heart muscle and the blood vessels around the heart, leading to heart failure.

Other Diseases and Conditions

Other diseases and conditions also can lead to heart failure, such as:
- Cardiomyopathy or heart muscle disease. Cardiomyopathy may be present at birth or caused by injury or infection.
- Heart valve disease. Problems with the heart valves may be present at birth or caused by infection, heart attack, or damage from heart disease.
- Arrhythmias or irregular heartbeats. These heart problems may be present at birth or caused by heart disease or heart defects.
- Congenital heart defects. These problems with the heart's structure are present at birth.

Other factors also can injure the heart muscle and lead to heart failure. Examples include:
- Treatments for cancer, such as radiation and chemotherapy
- Thyroid disorders (having either too much or too little thyroid hormone in the body)
- Alcohol abuse or cocaine and other illegal drug use
- HIV/AIDS
- Too much vitamin E

Heart damage from obstructive sleep apnea may worsen heart failure. Sleep apnea is a common disorder in which you have one or more pauses in breathing or shallow breaths while you sleep. Sleep apnea can deprive your heart of oxygen and increase its workload. Treating this sleep disorder might improve heart failure.

Heart failure is more common in:
- People who are 65 years old or older. Aging can weaken the heart muscle. Older people also may have had diseases for many years that led to heart failure. Heart failure is a leading cause of hospital stays among people on Medicare.
- African Americans. African Americans are more likely to have heart failure than people of other races. They're also more likely to have symptoms at a younger age, have more hospital visits due to heart failure, and die from heart failure.

- People who are overweight. Excess weight puts strain on the heart. Being overweight also increases your risk of heart disease and type 2 diabetes. These diseases can lead to heart failure.
- People who have had a heart attack.
- Men. Men have a higher rate of heart failure than women.

Children who have congenital heart defects also can develop heart failure. These defects occur if the heart, heart valves, or blood vessels near the heart don't form correctly while a baby is in the womb. Congenital heart defects can make the heart work harder. This weakens the heart muscle, which can lead to heart failure. Children don't have the same symptoms of heart failure or get the same treatments as adults.

Common Signs and Symptoms

The most common signs and symptoms of heart failure are:
- Shortness of breath or trouble breathing
- Fatigue (tiredness)
- Swelling in the ankles, feet, legs, abdomen, and veins in the neck

All of these symptoms are the result of fluid buildup in your body. When symptoms start, you may feel tired and short of breath after routine physical effort, like climbing stairs. As your heart grows weaker, symptoms get worse. You may begin to feel tired and short of breath after getting dressed or walking across the room. Some people have shortness of breath while lying flat.

Fluid buildup from heart failure also causes weight gain, frequent urination, and a cough that's worse at night and when you're lying down. This cough may be a sign of acute pulmonary edema. This is a condition in which too much fluid builds up in your lungs. The condition requires emergency treatment.

Diagnosis

Your doctor will diagnose heart failure based on your medical and family histories, a physical exam, and test results. The signs and symptoms of heart failure also are common in other conditions. Thus, your doctor will:

- Find out whether you have a disease or condition that can cause heart failure, such as coronary heart disease (CHD), high blood pressure, or diabetes
- Rule out other causes of your symptoms
- Find any damage to your heart and check how well your heart pumps blood

Early diagnosis and treatment can help people who have heart failure live longer, more active lives.

Medical and Family Histories

Your doctor will ask whether you or others in your family have or have had a disease or condition that can cause heart failure. Your doctor also will ask about your symptoms. He or she will want to know which symptoms you have, when they occur, how long you've had them, and how severe they are. Your answers will help show whether and how much your symptoms limit your daily routine.

Physical Exam

During the physical exam, your doctor will:

- Listen to your heart for sounds that aren't normal
- Listen to your lungs for the sounds of extra fluid buildup
- Look for swelling in your ankles, feet, legs, abdomen, and the veins in your neck

Diagnostic Tests

No single test can diagnose heart failure. If you have signs and symptoms of heart failure, your doctor may recommend one or more tests. Your doctor also may refer you to a cardiologist. A cardiologist is a doctor who specializes in diagnosing and treating heart diseases and conditions.

EKG (Electrocardiogram)

An EKG is a simple, painless test that detects and records the heart's electrical activity. The test shows how fast your heart is beating and its rhythm (steady or irregular). An EKG also records the strength and timing of electrical signals as they pass through your heart. An EKG may show whether the walls in your heart's pumping chambers are thicker than normal. Thicker walls can make it harder for your heart to pump blood. An EKG also can show signs of a previous or current heart attack.

Chest X Ray

A chest x ray takes pictures of the structures inside your chest, such as your heart, lungs, and blood vessels. This test can show whether your heart is enlarged, you have fluid in your lungs, or you have lung disease.

BNP Blood Test

This test checks the level of a hormone in your blood called BNP. The level of this hormone rises during heart failure.

Echocardiography

Echocardiography (echo) uses sound waves to create a moving picture of your heart. The test shows the size and shape of your heart and how well your heart chambers and valves work. Echo also can identify areas of poor blood flow to the heart, areas of heart muscle that aren't contracting normally, and heart muscle damage caused by lack of blood flow. Echo might be done before and after a stress test (see below). A stress echo can show how well blood is flowing through your heart. The test also can show how well your heart pumps blood when it beats.

Doppler Ultrasound

A Doppler ultrasound uses sound waves to measure the speed and direction of blood flow. This test often is done with echo to give a more complete picture of blood flow to the heart and lungs. Doctors often use Doppler ultrasound to help diagnose right-side heart failure.

Holter Monitor

A Holter monitor records your heart's electrical activity for a full 24- or 48-hour period, while you go about your normal daily routine. You wear small patches called electrodes on your chest. Wires connect the patches to a small, portable recorder. The recorder can be clipped to a belt, kept in a pocket, or hung around your neck.

Nuclear Heart Scan

A nuclear heart scan shows how well blood is flowing through your heart and how much blood is reaching your heart muscle. During a nuclear heart scan, a safe, radioactive substance called a tracer is injected into your bloodstream through a vein. The tracer travels to your heart and releases energy. Special cameras outside of your body detect the energy and use it to create pictures of your heart. A nuclear heart scan can show where the heart muscle is healthy and where it's damaged.

A positron emission tomography (PET) scan is a type of nuclear heart scan. It shows the level of chemical activity in areas of your heart. This test can help your doctor see whether enough blood is flowing to these areas. A PET scan can show blood flow problems that other tests might not detect.

Cardiac Catheterization

During cardiac catheterization, a long, thin, flexible tube called a catheter is put into a blood vessel in your arm, groin (upper thigh), or neck and threaded to your heart. This allows your doctor to look inside your coronary (heart) arteries. During this procedure, your doctor can check the pressure and blood flow in your heart chambers, collect blood samples, and use x rays to look at your coronary arteries.

Coronary Angiography

Coronary angiography usually is done with cardiac catheterization. A dye that can be seen on x ray is injected into your bloodstream through the tip of the catheter. The dye allows your doctor to see the flow of blood to your heart muscle. Angiography also shows how well your heart is pumping.

Stress Test

Some heart problems are easier to diagnose when your heart is working hard and beating fast. During stress testing, you exercise to make your heart work hard and beat fast. You may walk or run on a treadmill or pedal a bicycle. If you can't exercise, you may be given medicine to raise your heart rate. Heart tests, such as nuclear heart scanning and echo, often are done during stress testing.

Cardiac MRI

Cardiac MRI (magnetic resonance imaging) uses radio waves, magnets, and a computer to create pictures of your heart as it's beating. The test produces both still and moving pictures of your heart and major blood vessels. A cardiac MRI can show whether parts of your heart are damaged. Doctors also have used MRI in research studies to find early signs of heart failure, even before symptoms appear.

Thyroid Function Tests

Thyroid function tests show how well your thyroid gland is working. These tests include blood tests, imaging tests, and tests to stimulate the thyroid. Having too much or too little thyroid hormone in the blood can lead to heart failure.

Treatments

Early diagnosis and treatment can help people who have heart failure live longer, more active lives. Treatment for heart failure will depend on the type and stage of heart failure (the severity of the condition). The goals of treatment for all stages of heart failure include:
- Treating the condition's underlying cause, such as coronary heart disease (CHD), high blood pressure, or diabetes
- Reducing symptoms
- Stopping the heart failure from getting worse
- Increasing your lifespan and improving your quality of life

Treatments usually include lifestyle changes, medicines, and ongoing care. If you have severe heart failure, you also may need medical procedures or surgery.

Lifestyle Changes

Simple changes can help you feel better and control heart failure. The sooner you make these changes, the better off you'll likely be.

A Heart Healthy Diet

Following a heart healthy diet is an important part of managing heart failure. In fact, not having a proper diet can make heart failure worse. Ask your doctor and health care team to create an eating plan that works for you. A healthy diet includes a variety of vegetables and fruits. It also includes whole grains, fat-free or low-fat dairy products, and protein foods, such as lean meats, eggs, and poultry without skin, seafood, nuts, seeds, beans, and peas.

A healthy diet is low in sodium (salt) and solid fats (saturated fat and trans fatty acids). Too much salt can cause extra fluid to build up in your body, making heart failure worse. Saturated fat and trans fatty acids can cause unhealthy blood cholesterol levels, which are a risk factor for heart disease.

A healthy diet also is low in added sugars and refined grains. Refined grains come from processing whole grains, which results in a loss of nutrients (such as dietary fiber). Examples of refined grains include white rice and white bread.

A balanced, nutrient-rich diet can help your heart work better. Getting enough potassium is important for people who have heart failure. Some heart failure medicines deplete the potassium in your body. Lack of potassium can cause very rapid heart rhythms that can lead to sudden death.

Potassium is found in foods like white potatoes and sweet potatoes, greens (such as spinach), bananas, many dried fruits, and white beans and soybeans.

Talk with your health care team about getting the correct amount of potassium. Too much potassium also can be harmful.

Fluid Intake

It's important for people who have heart failure to drink the correct amounts and types of fluid. Drinking too much fluid can worsen heart failure. Also, if you have heart failure, you shouldn't drink alcohol. Talk with your doctor about what amounts and types of fluid you should have each day.

Other Lifestyle Changes

Taking steps to control risk factors for CHD, high blood pressure, and diabetes will help control heart failure. For example:

- Lose weight if you're overweight or obese. Work with your health care team to lose weight safely.
- Be physically active (as your doctor advises) to become more fit and stay as active as possible.
- Quit smoking and avoid using illegal drugs. Talk with your doctor about programs and products that can help you quit smoking. Also, try to avoid secondhand smoke. Smoking and drugs can worsen heart failure and harm your health.
- Get enough rest.

Medicines

Your doctor will prescribe medicines based on the type of heart failure you have, how severe it is, and your response to certain medicines. The following medicines are commonly used to treat heart failure:

- Diuretics (water or fluid pills) help reduce fluid buildup in your lungs and swelling in your feet and ankles.
- ACE inhibitors lower blood pressure and reduce strain on your heart. They also may reduce the risk of a future heart attack.
- Aldosterone antagonists trigger the body to get rid of salt and water through urine. This lowers the volume of blood that the heart must pump.
- Angiotensin receptor blockers relax your blood vessels and lower blood pressure to decrease your heart's workload.
- Beta blockers slow your heart rate and lower your blood pressure to decrease your heart's workload.
- Isosorbide dinitrate/hydralazine hydrochloride helps relax your blood vessels so your heart doesn't work as hard to pump blood. Studies have shown that this medicine can reduce the risk of death in African Americans. More studies are needed to find out whether this medicine will benefit other racial groups.
- Digoxin makes the heart beat stronger and pump more blood.

Ongoing Care

You should watch for signs that heart failure is getting worse. For example, weight gain may mean that fluids are building up in your body. Ask your doctor how often you should check your weight and when to report weight changes.

Getting medical care for other related conditions is important. If you have diabetes or high blood pressure, work with your health care team to control these conditions. Have your blood sugar level and blood pressure checked. Talk with your doctor about when you should have tests and how often to take measurements at home.

Try to avoid respiratory infections like the flu and pneumonia. Talk with your doctor or nurse about getting flu and pneumonia vaccines.

Many people who have severe heart failure may need treatment in a hospital from time to time. Your doctor may recommend oxygen therapy (oxygen given through nasal prongs or a mask). Oxygen therapy can be given in a hospital or at home.

Medical Procedures and Surgery

As heart failure worsens, lifestyle changes and medicines may no longer control your symptoms. You may need a medical procedure or surgery. If you have heart damage and severe heart failure symptoms, your doctor might recommend a cardiac resynchronization therapy (CRT) device or an implantable cardioverter defibrillator (ICD).

In heart failure, the right and left sides of the heart may no longer contract at the same time. This disrupts the heart's pumping. To correct this problem, your doctor might implant a CRT device (a type of pacemaker) near your heart. This device helps both sides of your heart contract at the same time, which can decrease heart failure symptoms.

Some people who have heart failure have very rapid, irregular heartbeats. Without treatment, these heartbeats can cause sudden cardiac arrest. Your doctor might implant an ICD near your heart to solve this problem. An ICD checks your heart rate and uses electrical pulses to correct irregular heart rhythms.

People who have severe heart failure symptoms at rest, despite other treatments, may need:

- A mechanical heart pump, such as a left ventricular assist device. This device helps pump blood from the heart to the rest of the body. You may use a heart pump until you have surgery or as a long-term treatment.
- Heart transplant. A heart transplant is an operation in which a person's diseased heart is replaced with a healthy heart from a deceased donor. Heart transplants are done as a life-saving measure for end-stage heart failure when medical treatment and less drastic surgery have failed.
- Experimental treatments. Studies are under way to find new and better ways to treat heart failure.

Ongoing Research

Researchers continue to learn more about heart failure and how to treat it. As a result, treatments are getting better. If you have heart failure, you may want to consider taking part in research studies called clinical trials.

These studies offer care from experts and the chance to help advance heart failure knowledge and treatment.

If you have heart failure, you may also want to take part in a heart failure registry. The registry tracks the course of disease and treatment in large numbers of people. These data help research move forward. You may help yourself and others by taking part. Talk with your health care team to learn more.

Prevention

You can take steps to prevent heart failure. The sooner you start, the better your chances of preventing or delaying the condition. If you have a healthy heart, you can take action to prevent heart disease and heart failure. To reduce your risk of heart disease:

- Follow a healthy diet. A healthy diet includes a variety of vegetables and fruits. It also includes whole grains, fat-free or low-fat dairy products, and protein foods. A healthy diet is low in sodium (salt), added sugars, solid fats, and refined grains.
- If you smoke, make an effort to quit. Talk with your doctor about programs and products that can help you quit smoking. Also, try to avoid secondhand smoke.
- If you're overweight or obese, try to lose weight. Work with your health care team to create a reasonable weight-loss plan.
- Be physically active. People gain health benefits from as little as 60 minutes of moderate-intensity aerobic activity per week. The more active you are, the more you will benefit.
- Avoid using illegal drugs.

For People Who Are at High Risk for Heart Failure

Even if you're at high risk for heart failure, you can take steps to reduce your risk. People at high risk include those who have coronary heart disease, high blood pressure, or diabetes.

- Follow all of the steps listed above. Talk with your doctor about what types and amounts of physical activity are safe for you.
- Treat and control any conditions that can cause heart failure. Take medicines as your doctor prescribes.
- Avoid drinking alcohol.

- See your doctor for ongoing care.

For People Who Have Heart Damage but No Signs of Heart Failure

If you have heart damage but no signs of heart failure, you can still reduce your risk of developing the condition. In addition to the steps above, take your medicines as prescribed to reduce your heart's workload.

Living with Heart Failure

Currently, heart failure has no cure. You'll likely have to take medicine and follow a treatment plan for the rest of your life. Despite treatment, symptoms may get worse over time. You may not be able to do many of the things that you did before you had heart failure. However, if you take all the steps your doctor recommends, you can stay healthier longer. Researchers also might find new treatments that can help you in the future.

Follow Your Treatment Plan

Treatment can relieve your symptoms and make daily activities easier. It also can reduce the chance that you'll have to go to the hospital. Thus, it's important that you follow your treatment plan.

- Take your medicines as your doctor prescribes. If you have side effects from any of your medicines, tell your doctor. He or she might adjust the dose or type of medicine you take to relieve side effects.
- Make all of the lifestyle changes that your doctor recommends.
- Get advice from your doctor about how active you can and should be. This includes advice on daily activities, work, leisure time, sex, and exercise. Your level of activity will depend on the stage of your heart failure (how severe it is).
- Keep all of your medical appointments, including visits to the doctor and appointments to get tests and lab work. Your doctor needs the results of these tests to adjust your medicine doses and help you avoid harmful side effects.

Take Steps to Prevent Heart Failure from Getting Worse

Certain actions can worsen your heart failure, such as:
- Forgetting to take your medicines

- Not following your diet (for example, eating salty foods)
- Drinking alcohol

These actions can lead to a hospital stay. If you have trouble following your diet, talk with your doctor. He or she can help arrange for a dietitian to work with you. Avoid drinking alcohol.

People who have heart failure often have other serious conditions that require ongoing treatment. If you have other serious conditions, you're likely taking medicines for them as well as for heart failure. Taking more than one medicine raises the risk of side effects and other problems. Make sure your doctors and your pharmacist have a complete list of all of the medicines and over-the-counter products that you're taking.

Tell your doctor right away about any problems with your medicines. Also, talk with your doctor before taking any new medicine prescribed by another doctor or any new over-the-counter medicines or herbal supplements.

Try to avoid respiratory infections like the flu and pneumonia. Ask your doctor or nurse about getting flu and pneumonia vaccines.

Plan Ahead

If you have heart failure, it's important to know:
- When to seek help. Ask your doctor when to make an office visit or get emergency care.
- Phone numbers for your doctor and hospital.
- Directions to your doctor's office and hospital and people who can take you there.
- A list of medicines you're taking.

Emotional Issues and Support

Living with heart failure may cause fear, anxiety, depression, and stress. Talk about how you feel with your health care team. Talking to a professional counselor also can help. If you're very depressed, your doctor may recommend medicines or other treatments that can improve your quality of life.

Joining a patient support group may help you adjust to living with heart failure. You can see how other people who have the same symptoms have coped with them. Talk with your doctor about local support groups or check with an area medical center.

Support from family and friends also can help relieve stress and anxiety. Let your loved ones know how you feel and what they can do to help you.

STROKE

Stroke is the number three cause of death in women, and the number four cause of death in men. Lifestyle changes that can reduce your risk of stroke, according to the Mayo Clinic, include quitting smoking, losing excess weight, exercising, and eating a healthy diet.

3

Cancer

Overall cancer death rates continue to decline in the United States among both men and women, among all major racial and ethnic groups, and for all of the most common cancer sites, including lung, colon and rectum, female breast, and prostate. The decline in overall cancer death rates continues a trend that began in the early 1990s. Death rates decreased by 1.8 percent per year among men and by 1.4 percent per year among women. Death rates among children up to 14 years of age also continued to decrease by 1.8 percent per year.

During 2000 through 2009, death rates among men decreased for 10 of the 17 most common cancers (lung, prostate, colon and rectum, leukemia, non-Hodgkin lymphoma, kidney, stomach, myeloma, oral cavity and pharynx, and larynx) and increased for melanoma of the skin and cancers of the pancreas and liver. During the same 10-year period, death rates among women decreased for 15 of the 18 most common cancers (lung, breast, colon and rectum, ovary, leukemia, non-Hodgkin lymphoma, brain and other nervous system, myeloma, kidney, stomach, cervix, bladder, esophagus, oral cavity and pharynx, and gallbladder) and increased for cancers of the pancreas, liver, and uterus.

Lung cancer is the cancer responsible for the most deaths in both men and women. Women are also affected greatly by breast and colorectal cancers.

Cancer is the name given to a collection of related diseases. In all types of cancer, some of the body's cells begin to divide without stopping and spread into surrounding tissues. Cancer can start almost anywhere in the human body, which is made up of trillions of cells. Normally, human cells grow and divide to form new cells as the body needs them. When cells grow old or become damaged, they die, and new cells take their place.

When cancer develops, however, this orderly process breaks down. As cells become more and more abnormal, old or damaged cells survive when they should die, and new cells form when they are not needed. These extra cells can divide without stopping and may form growths called tumors.

Many cancers form solid tumors, which are masses of tissue. Cancers of the blood, such as leukemias, generally do not form solid tumors. Cancerous tumors are malignant, which means they can spread into, or invade, nearby tissues. In addition, as these tumors grow, some cancer cells can break off and travel to distant places in the body through the blood or the lymph system and form new tumors far from the original tumor.

Unlike malignant tumors, benign tumors do not spread into, or invade, nearby tissues. Benign tumors can sometimes be quite large, however. When removed, they usually don't grow back, whereas malignant tumors sometimes do. Unlike most benign tumors elsewhere in the body, benign brain tumors can be life threatening.

Cancer cells differ from normal cells in many ways that allow them to grow out of control and become invasive. One important difference is that cancer cells are less specialized than normal cells. That is, whereas normal cells mature into very distinct cell types with specific functions, cancer cells do not. This is one reason that, unlike normal cells, cancer cells continue to divide without stopping.

In addition, cancer cells are able to ignore signals that normally tell cells to stop dividing or that begin a process known as programmed cell death, or apoptosis, which the body uses to get rid of unneeded cells.

Cancer cells may be able to influence the normal cells, molecules, and blood vessels that surround and feed a tumor—an area known as the microenvironment. For instance, cancer cells can induce nearby normal cells to form blood vessels that supply tumors with oxygen and nutrients, which they need to grow. These blood vessels also remove waste products from tumors.

Cancer cells are also often able to evade the immune system, a network of organs, tissues, and specialized cells that protects the body from infections and other conditions. Although the immune system normally removes damaged or abnormal cells from the body, some cancer cells are able to "hide" from the immune system.

Tumors can also use the immune system to stay alive and grow. For example, with the help of certain immune system cells that normally prevent a runaway immune response, cancer cells can actually keep the immune system from killing cancer cells.

WHAT CAUSES CANCER?

Cancer is a genetic disease—that is, it is caused by changes to genes that control the way our cells function, especially how they grow and divide. Genetic changes that cause cancer can be inherited from our parents. They can also arise during a person's lifetime as a result of errors that occur as cells divide or because of damage to DNA caused by certain environmental exposures. Cancer-causing environmental exposures include substances, such as the chemicals in tobacco smoke, and radiation, such as ultraviolet rays from the sun.

Each person's cancer has a unique combination of genetic changes. As the cancer continues to grow, additional changes will occur. Even within the same tumor, different cells may have different genetic changes.

In general, cancer cells have more genetic changes, such as mutations in DNA, than normal cells. Some of these changes may have nothing to do with the cancer; they may be the result of the cancer, rather than its cause.

The genetic changes that contribute to cancer tend to affect three main types of genes—proto-oncogenes, tumor suppressor genes, and DNA repair genes. These changes are sometimes called "drivers" of cancer.

Proto-oncogenes are involved in normal cell growth and division. However, when these genes are altered in certain ways or are more active than normal, they may become cancer-causing genes (or oncogenes), allowing cells to grow and survive when they should not.

Tumor suppressor genes are also involved in controlling cell growth and division. Cells with certain alterations in tumor suppressor genes may divide in an uncontrolled manner.

DNA repair genes are involved in fixing damaged DNA. Cells with mutations in these genes tend to develop additional mutations in other genes. Together, these mutations may cause the cells to become cancerous.

As scientists have learned more about the molecular changes that lead to cancer, they have found that certain mutations commonly occur in many types of cancer. Because of this, cancers are sometimes characterized by the types of genetic alterations that are believed to be driving them, not just by where they develop in the body and how the cancer cells look under the microscope.

WHEN CANCER SPREADS

A cancer that has spread from the place where it first started to another place in the body is called metastatic cancer. The process by which cancer cells spread to other parts of the body is called metastasis. Metastatic cancer has the same name and the same type of cancer cells as the original, or primary, cancer. For example, breast cancer that spreads to and forms a metastatic tumor in the lung is metastatic breast cancer, not lung cancer.

Under a microscope, metastatic cancer cells generally look the same as cells of the original cancer. Moreover, metastatic cancer cells and cells of the original cancer usually have some molecular features in common, such as the presence of specific chromosome changes.

Treatment may help prolong the lives of some people with metastatic cancer. In general, though, the primary goal of treatments for metastatic cancer is to control the growth of the cancer or to relieve symptoms caused by it. Metastatic tumors can cause severe damage to how the body functions, and most people who die of cancer die of metastatic disease.

Not every change in the body's tissues is cancer. Some tissue changes may develop into cancer if they are not treated, however. Here are some examples of tissue changes that are not cancer but, in some cases, are monitored:

- Hyperplasia occurs when cells within a tissue divide faster than normal and extra cells build up, or proliferate. However, the cells and the way the tissue is organized look normal under a microscope. Hyperplasia can be caused by several factors or conditions, including chronic irritation.
- Dysplasia is a more serious condition than hyperplasia. In dysplasia, there is also a buildup of extra cells. But the cells look abnormal and there are changes in how the tissue is organized. In general, the more abnormal the cells and tissue look, the greater the chance that cancer will form.

Some types of dysplasia may need to be monitored or treated. An example of dysplasia is an abnormal mole (called a dysplastic nevus) that forms on the skin. A dysplastic nevus can turn into melanoma, although most do not.

An even more serious condition is carcinoma in situ. Although it is sometimes called cancer, carcinoma in situ is not cancer because the abnormal cells do not spread beyond the original tissue. That is, they do not invade nearby tissue the way that cancer cells do. But, because some carcinomas in situ may become cancer, they are usually treated.

TYPES OF CANCER

There are more than 100 types of cancer. Types of cancer are usually named for the organs or tissues where the cancers form. For example, lung cancer starts in cells of the lung, and brain cancer starts in cells of the brain. Cancers also may be described by the type of cell that formed them, such as an epithelial cell or a squamous cell. Here are some categories of cancers that begin in specific types of cells:

Carcinoma

Carcinomas are the most common type of cancer. They are formed by epithelial cells, which are the cells that cover the inside and outside surfaces of the body. There are many types of epithelial cells, which often have a column-like shape when viewed under a microscope. Carcinomas that begin in different epithelial cell types have specific names:

Adenocarcinoma is a cancer that forms in epithelial cells that produce fluids or mucus. Tissues with this type of epithelial cell are sometimes called glandular tissues. Most cancers of the breast, colon, and prostate are adenocarcinomas.

Basal cell carcinoma is a cancer that begins in the lower or basal (base) layer of the epidermis, which is a person's outer layer of skin.

Squamous cell carcinoma is a cancer that forms in squamous cells, which are epithelial cells that lie just beneath the outer surface of the skin. Squamous cells also line many other organs, including the stomach, intestines, lungs, bladder, and kidneys. Squamous cells look flat, like fish scales, when viewed under a microscope. Squamous cell carcinomas are sometimes called epidermoid carcinomas.

Transitional cell carcinoma is a cancer that forms in a type of epithelial tissue called transitional epithelium, or urothelium. This tissue, which is made up of many layers of epithelial cells that can get bigger and smaller, is found in the linings of the bladder, ureters, and part of the kidneys (renal pelvis), and a few other organs. Some cancers of the bladder, ureters, and kidneys are transitional cell carcinomas.

Sarcoma

Sarcomas are cancers that form in bone and soft tissues, including muscle, fat, blood vessels, lymph vessels, and fibrous tissue (such as tendons and ligaments).

Osteosarcoma is the most common cancer of bone. The most common types of soft tissue sarcoma are leiomyosarcoma, Kaposi sarcoma, malignant fibrous histiocytoma, liposarcoma, and dermatofibrosarcoma protuberans.

Leukemia

Cancers that begin in the blood-forming tissue of the bone marrow are called leukemias. These cancers do not form solid tumors. Instead, large numbers of abnormal white blood cells (leukemia cells and leukemic blast cells) build up in the blood and bone marrow, crowding out normal blood cells. The low level of normal blood cells can make it harder for the body to get oxygen to its tissues, control bleeding, or fight infections. There are four common types of leukemia, which are grouped based on how quickly the disease gets worse (acute or chronic) and on the type of blood cell the cancer starts in (lymphoblastic or myeloid).

Lymphoma

Lymphoma is cancer that begins in lymphocytes (T cells or B cells). These are disease-fighting white blood cells that are part of the immune system. In lymphoma, abnormal lymphocytes build up in lymph nodes and lymph vessels, as well as in other organs of the body. There are two main types of lymphoma:

- Hodgkin lymphoma – People with this disease have abnormal lymphocytes that are called Reed-Sternberg cells. These cells usually form from B cells.

- Non-Hodgkin lymphoma – This is a large group of cancers that start in lymphocytes. The cancers can grow quickly or slowly and can form from B cells or T cells.

Multiple Myeloma

Multiple myeloma is cancer that begins in plasma cells, another type of immune cell. The abnormal plasma cells, called myeloma cells, build up in the bone marrow and form tumors in bones all through the body. Multiple myeloma is also called plasma cell myeloma and Kahler disease.

Melanoma

Melanoma is cancer that begins in cells that become melanocytes, which are specialized cells that make melanin (the pigment that gives skin its color). Most melanomas form on the skin, but melanomas can also form in other pigmented tissues, such as the eye.

Brain and Spinal Cord Tumors

There are different types of brain and spinal cord tumors. These tumors are named based on the type of cell in which they formed and where the tumor first formed in the central nervous system. For example, an astrocytic tumor begins in star-shaped brain cells called astrocytes, which help keep nerve cells healthy. Brain tumors can be benign (not cancer) or malignant (cancer).

Other Types of Tumors

Germ Cell Tumors

Germ cell tumors are a type of tumor that begins in the cells that give rise to sperm or eggs. These tumors can occur almost anywhere in the body and can be either benign or malignant.

Neuroendocrine Tumors

Neuroendocrine tumors form from cells that release hormones into the blood in response to a signal from the nervous system. These tumors, which may make higher-than-normal amounts of hormones, can cause many different symptoms. Neuroendocrine tumors may be benign or malignant.

Carcinoid Tumors

Carcinoid tumors are a type of neuroendocrine tumor. They are slow-growing tumors that are usually found in the gastrointestinal system (most often in the rectum and small intestine). Carcinoid tumors may spread to the liver or other sites in the body, and they may secrete substances such as serotonin or prostaglandins, causing carcinoid syndrome.

TREATMENTS

Your medical team has multiple options for treating your cancer ranging from immunotherapy—using the immune system to fight the cancer—to chemotherapy, radiation, targeted therapies and surgery.

Chemotherapy

Chemotherapy (also called chemo) is a type of cancer treatment that uses drugs to destroy cancer cells. Chemotherapy works by stopping or slowing the growth of cancer cells, which grow and divide quickly. But it can also harm healthy cells that divide quickly, such as those that line your mouth and intestines or cause your hair to grow. Damage to healthy cells may cause side effects. Often, side effects get better or go away after chemotherapy is over. Depending on your type of cancer and how advanced it is, chemotherapy can:

- Cure cancer—when chemotherapy destroys cancer cells to the point that your doctor can no longer detect them in your body and they will not grow back.
- Control cancer—when chemotherapy keeps cancer from spreading, slows its growth, or destroys cancer cells that have spread to other parts of your body.

- Ease cancer symptoms (also called palliative care)—when chemotherapy shrinks tumors that are causing pain or pressure.

Sometimes, chemotherapy is used as the only cancer treatment. But more often, you will get chemotherapy along with surgery, radiation therapy, or biological therapy. Chemotherapy can:

- Make a tumor smaller before surgery or radiation therapy. This is called neo-adjuvant chemotherapy.
- Destroy cancer cells that may remain after surgery or radiation therapy. This is called adjuvant chemotherapy.
- Help radiation therapy and biological therapy work better.
- Destroy cancer cells that have come back (recurrent cancer) or spread to other parts of your body (metastatic cancer).

This choice depends on:

- The type of cancer you have. Some types of chemotherapy drugs are used for many types of cancer. Other drugs are used for just one or two types of cancer.
- Whether you have had chemotherapy before.
- Whether you have other health problems, such as diabetes or heart disease.

You may receive chemotherapy during a hospital stay, at home, or in a doctor's office, clinic, or outpatient unit in a hospital (which means you do not have to stay overnight). No matter where you go for chemotherapy, your doctor and nurse will watch for side effects and make any needed drug changes.

Treatment schedules for chemotherapy vary widely. How often and how long you get chemotherapy depends on:

- Your type of cancer and how advanced it is
- The goals of treatment (whether chemotherapy is used to cure your cancer, control its growth, or ease the symptoms)
- The type of chemotherapy
- How your body reacts to chemotherapy

You may receive chemotherapy in cycles. A cycle is a period of chemotherapy treatment followed by a period of rest. For instance, you might receive 1 week of chemotherapy followed by 3 weeks of rest. These 4 weeks make up one cycle. The rest period gives your body a chance to build new healthy cells.

It is not good to skip a chemotherapy treatment. But sometimes your doctor or nurse may change your chemotherapy schedule. This can be due to side affects you are having. If this happens, your doctor or nurse will explain what to do and when to start treatment again.

Chemotherapy may be given in many ways.

- Injection. The chemotherapy is given by a shot in a muscle in your arm, thigh, or hip, or right under the skin in the fatty part of your arm, leg, or belly.
- Intra-arterial (IA). The chemotherapy goes directly into the artery that is feeding the cancer.
- Intraperitoneal (IP). The chemotherapy goes directly into the peritoneal cavity (the area that contains organs such as your intestines, stomach, liver, and ovaries).
- Intravenous (IV). The chemotherapy goes directly into a vein.
- Topical. The chemotherapy comes in a cream that you rub onto your skin.
- Oral. The chemotherapy comes in pills, capsules, or liquids that you swallow.

Chemotherapy affects people in different ways. How you feel depends on how healthy you are before treatment, your type of cancer, how advanced it is, the kind of chemotherapy you are getting, and the dose. Doctors and nurses cannot know for certain how you will feel during chemotherapy. Some people do not feel well right after chemotherapy. The most common side effect is fatigue, feeling exhausted and worn out. You can prepare for fatigue by:

- Asking someone to drive you to and from chemotherapy
- Planning time to rest on the day of and day after chemotherapy
- Getting help with meals and childcare the day of and at least 1 day after chemotherapy

There are many ways you can help manage chemotherapy side effects.

Many people can work during chemotherapy, as long as they match their schedule to how they feel. Whether or not you can work may depend on what kind of work you do. If your job allows, you may want to see if you can work part-time or work from home on days you do not feel well. Many employers are required by law to change your work schedule to meet your needs during cancer treatment. Talk with your employer about ways to adjust your work during chemotherapy. You can learn more about these laws by talking with a social worker.

Radiation

Radiation therapy uses high-energy radiation to kill cancer cells by damaging their DNA.

Radiation therapy can damage normal cells as well as cancer cells. Therefore, treatment must be carefully planned to minimize side effects.

The radiation used for cancer treatment may come from a machine outside the body, or it may come from radioactive material placed in the body near tumor cells or injected into the bloodstream.

A patient may receive radiation therapy before, during, or after surgery, depending on the type of cancer being treated.

Some patients receive radiation therapy alone, and some receive radiation therapy in combination with chemotherapy.

Radiation therapy uses high-energy radiation to shrink tumors and kill cancer cells. X-rays, gamma rays, and charged particles are types of radiation used for cancer treatment. The radiation may be delivered by a machine outside the body (external-beam radiation therapy), or it may come from radioactive material placed in the body near cancer cells (internal radiation therapy, also called brachytherapy).

Systemic radiation therapy uses radioactive substances, such as radioactive iodine, that travel in the blood to kill cancer cells. About half of all cancer patients receive some type of radiation therapy sometime during the course of their treatment.

Radiation therapy kills cancer cells by damaging their DNA (the molecules inside cells that carry genetic information and pass it from one generation to the next). Radiation therapy can either damage DNA directly or create charged particles (free radicals) within the cells that can in turn damage the DNA. Cancer cells whose DNA is damaged beyond repair stop dividing or die. When the damaged cells die, they are broken down and eliminated by the body's natural processes.

Radiation therapy can also damage normal cells, leading to side effects. Doctors take potential damage to normal cells into account when planning a course of radiation therapy. The amount of radiation that normal tissue can safely receive is known for all parts of the body. Doctors use this information to help them decide where to aim radiation during treatment.

Radiation therapy is sometimes given with curative intent (that is, with the hope that the treatment will cure a cancer, either by eliminating a tumor, preventing cancer recurrence, or both). In such cases, radiation therapy may be used alone or in combination with surgery, chemotherapy, or both.

Radiation therapy may also be given with palliative intent. Palliative treatments are not intended to cure. Instead, they relieve symptoms and reduce the suffering caused by cancer.

Some examples of palliative radiation therapy are:

Radiation given to the brain to shrink tumors formed from cancer cells that have spread to the brain from another part of the body (metastases).

Radiation given to shrink a tumor that is pressing on the spine or growing within a bone, which can cause pain.

Radiation given to shrink a tumor near the esophagus, which can interfere with a patient's ability to eat and drink.

A radiation oncologist develops a patient's treatment plan through a process called treatment planning, which begins with simulation. During simulation, detailed imaging scans show the location of a patient's tumor and the normal areas around it. These scans are usually computed tomography (CT) scans, but they can also include magnetic resonance imaging (MRI), positron emission tomography (PET), and ultrasound scans.

During simulation and daily treatments, it is necessary to ensure that the patient will be in exactly the same position every day relative to the machine delivering the treatment or doing the imaging. Body molds, head masks, or other devices may be constructed for an individual patient to make it easier for a patient to stay still. Temporary skin marks and even tattoos are used to help with precise patient positioning.

After simulation, the radiation oncologist then determines the exact area that will be treated, the total radiation dose that will be delivered to the tumor, how much dose will be allowed for the normal tissues around the tumor, and the safest angles (paths) for radiation delivery. The area selected for treatment usually includes the whole tumor plus a small amount of normal tissue surrounding the tumor. The normal tissue is treated for two main reasons:

To take into account body movement from breathing and normal movement of the organs within the body, which can change the location of a tumor between treatments.

To reduce the likelihood of tumor recurrence from cancer cells that have spread to the normal tissue next to the tumor (called microscopic local spread).

Systemic radiation therapy

In systemic radiation therapy, a patient swallows or receives an injection of a radioactive substance, such as radioactive iodine or a radioactive substance bound to a monoclonal antibody. Radioactive iodine is a type of systemic radiation therapy commonly used to help treat some types of thyroid cancer. Thyroid cells naturally take up radioactive iodine.

For systemic radiation therapy for some other types of cancer, a monoclonal antibody helps target the radioactive substance to the right place. The antibody joined to the radioactive substance travels through the blood, locating and killing tumor cells. Many other systemic radiation therapy drugs are in clinical trials for different cancer types.

Patients who receive most types of external-beam radiation therapy usually have to travel to the hospital or an outpatient facility up to 5 days a week for several weeks. One dose (a single fraction) of the total planned dose of radiation is given each day. Occasionally, two treatments a day are given.

A patient may receive radiation therapy before, during, or after surgery. Some patients may receive radiation therapy alone, without surgery or other treatments. Some patients may receive radiation therapy and chemotherapy at the same time. The timing of radiation therapy depends on the type of cancer being treated and the goal of treatment (cure or palliation).

The combination of chemotherapy and radiation therapy given at the same time is sometimes called chemoradiation or radiochemotherapy. For some types of cancer, the combination of chemotherapy and radiation therapy may kill more cancer cells (increasing the likelihood of a cure), but it can also cause more side effects.

After cancer treatment, patients receive regular follow-up care from their oncologists to monitor their health and to check for possible cancer recurrence.

Radiation therapy can cause both early (acute) and late (chronic) side effects. Acute side effects occur during treatment, and chronic side effects occur months or even years after treatment ends. The side effects that develop depend on the area of the body being treated, the dose given per day, the total dose given, the patient's general medical condition, and other treatments given at the same time.

Fatigue is a common side effect of radiation therapy regardless of which part of the body is treated. Nausea with or without vomiting is common when the abdomen is treated and occurs sometimes when the brain is treated. Medications are available to help prevent or treat nausea and vomiting during treatment.

Doctors and other scientists are conducting research studies called clinical trials to learn how to use radiation therapy to treat cancer more safely and effectively. Clinical trials allow researchers to examine the effectiveness of new treatments in comparison with standard ones, as well as to compare the side effects of the treatments.

Researchers are working on improving image-guided radiation so that it provides real-time imaging of the tumor target during treatment. Real-time imaging could help compensate for normal movement of the internal organs from breathing and for changes in tumor size during treatment.

Targeted Cancer Therapies

Targeted cancer therapies are drugs or other substances that interfere with specific molecules involved in cancer cell growth and survival. Traditional chemotherapy drugs, by contrast, act against all actively dividing cells.

Targeted cancer therapies that have been approved for use against specific cancers include agents that prevent cell growth signaling, interfere with tumor blood vessel development, promote the death of cancer cells, stimulate the immune system to destroy cancer cells, and deliver toxic drugs to cancer cells.

Targeted cancer therapies are sometimes called "molecularly targeted drugs," "molecularly targeted therapies," "precision medicines," or similar names. Targeted therapies differ from standard chemotherapy in several ways:

- Targeted therapies act on specific molecular targets that are associated with cancer, whereas most standard chemotherapies act on all rapidly dividing normal and cancerous cells.
- Targeted therapies are deliberately chosen or designed to interact with their target, whereas many standard chemotherapies were identified because they kill cells.
- Targeted therapies are often cytostatic (that is, they block tumor cell proliferation), whereas standard chemotherapy agents are cytotoxic (that is, they kill tumor cells).

Targeted therapies are currently the focus of much anticancer drug development. They are a cornerstone of precision medicine, a form of medicine that uses information about a person's genes and proteins to prevent, diagnose, and treat disease.

Many targeted cancer therapies have been approved by the Food and Drug Administration (FDA) to treat specific types of cancer. Others are being studied in clinical trials, and many more are in preclinical testing (research studies with animals).

The development of targeted therapies requires the identification of good targets—that is, targets that play a key role in cancer cell growth and survival. (It is for this reason that targeted therapies are sometimes referred to as the product of "rational" drug design.)

One approach to identify potential targets is to compare the amounts of individual proteins in cancer cells with those in normal cells. Proteins that are present in cancer cells but not normal cells or that are more abundant in cancer cells would be potential targets, especially if they are known to be involved in cell growth or survival. Another approach to identify potential targets is to determine whether cancer cells produce mutant (altered) proteins that drive cancer progression.

Researchers also look for abnormalities in chromosomes that are present in cancer cells but not in normal cells. Sometimes these chromosome abnormalities result in the creation of a fusion gene (a gene that incorporates parts of two different genes) whose product, called a fusion protein, may drive cancer development. Such fusion proteins are potential targets for targeted cancer therapies.

Most targeted therapies are either small molecules or monoclonal antibodies. Small-molecule compounds are typically developed for targets that are located inside the cell because such agents are able to enter cells relatively easily. Monoclonal antibodies are relatively large and generally cannot enter cells, so they are used only for targets that are outside cells or on the cell surface.

Many different targeted therapies have been approved for use in cancer treatment. These therapies include hormone therapies, signal transduction inhibitors, gene expression modulator, apoptosis inducer, angiogenesis inhibitor, immunotherapies, and toxin delivery molecules.

- Hormone therapies slow or stop the growth of hormone-sensitive tumors, which require certain hormones to grow. Hormone therapies act by preventing the body from producing the hormones or by interfering with the action of the hormones. Hormone therapies have been approved for both breast cancer and prostate cancer.

- Signal transduction inhibitors block the activities of molecules that participate in signal transduction, the process by which a cell responds to signals from its environment. During this process, once a cell has received a specific signal, the signal is relayed within the cell through a series of biochemical reactions that ultimately produce the appropriate response(s). In some cancers, the malignant cells are stimulated to divide continuously without being prompted to do so by external growth factors. Signal transduction inhibitors interfere with this inappropriate signaling.
- Gene expression modulators modify the function of proteins that play a role in controlling gene expression.
- Apoptosis inducers cause cancer cells to undergo a process of controlled cell death called apoptosis. Apoptosis is one method the body uses to get rid of unneeded or abnormal cells, but cancer cells have strategies to avoid apoptosis. Apoptosis inducers can get around these strategies to cause the death of cancer cells.
- Angiogenesis inhibitors block the growth of new blood vessels to tumors (a process called tumor angiogenesis). A blood supply is necessary for tumors to grow beyond a certain size because blood provides the oxygen and nutrients that tumors need for continued growth. Treatments that interfere with angiogenesis may block tumor growth. Some targeted therapies that inhibit angiogenesis interfere with the action of vascular endothelial growth factor (VEGF), a substance that stimulates new blood vessel formation. Other angiogenesis inhibitors target other molecules that stimulate new blood vessel growth.
- Immunotherapies trigger the immune system to destroy cancer cells. Some immunotherapies are monoclonal antibodies that recognize specific molecules on the surface of cancer cells. Binding of the monoclonal antibody to the target molecule results in the immune destruction of cells that express that target molecule. Other monoclonal antibodies bind to certain immune cells to help these cells better kill cancer cells.
- Monoclonal antibodies that deliver toxic molecules can cause the death of cancer cells specifically. Once the antibody has bound to its target cell, the toxic molecule that is linked to the antibody—such as a radioactive substance or a poisonous chemical—is taken up by the cell, ultimately killing that cell. The toxin will not affect cells that lack the target for the antibody—i.e., the vast majority of cells in the body.

Sometimes, a patient is a candidate for a targeted therapy only if he or she meets specific criteria (for example, their cancer did not respond to other therapies, has spread, or is inoperable). These criteria are set by the FDA when it approves a specific targeted therapy.

Targeted therapies do have some limitations. One is that cancer cells can become resistant to them. Resistance can occur in two ways: the target itself changes through mutation so that the targeted therapy no longer interacts well with it, and/or the tumor finds a new pathway to achieve tumor growth that does not depend on the target. Another approach is to use a targeted therapy in combination with one or more traditional chemotherapy drugs.

Scientists had expected that targeted cancer therapies would be less toxic than traditional chemotherapy drugs because cancer cells are more dependent on the targets than are normal cells. However, targeted cancer therapies can have substantial side effects. The most common side effects seen with targeted therapies are diarrhea and liver problems, such as hepatitis and elevated liver enzymes.   Other side effects seen with targeted therapies include:

- Skin problems (acneiform rash, dry skin, nail changes, hair depigmentation)
- Problems with blood clotting and wound healing
- High blood pressure
- Gastrointestinal perforation (a rare side effect of some targeted therapies)

The few targeted therapies that are approved for use in children can have different side effects in children than in adults, including immunosuppression and impaired sperm production.

CANCER IN CHILDREN AND ADOLESCENTS

Childhood cancer is the leading cause of disease-related death among children and adolescents (ages 1 to 19 years) in the United States, although cancer among children is rare.

The causes of childhood cancer are not well understood.

Survival rates for most childhood cancers vary widely across cancer types. Survival rates for some cancers have improved in recent years, and, overall, more than 80 percent of children and adolescents who are diagnosed with cancer live at least 5 years after their diagnosis. However, for some childhood cancer types, survival rates remain low.

Children and adolescents who have been treated for cancer need regular follow-up care for the rest of their lives because they are at risk of late side effects that can occur many years later, including second cancers.

Although cancer in children is rare, it is the leading cause of death by disease past infancy among children in the United States. In 2014, it is estimated that 15,780 children and adolescents ages 0 to 19 years will be diagnosed with cancer and 1,960 will die of the disease in the United States.

The most common types of cancer diagnosed in children and adolescents are leukemia, brain and central nervous system tumors, lymphoma, rhabdomyosarcoma, neuroblastoma, Wilms tumor, bone cancer, and gonadal (testicular and ovarian) germ cell tumors.

There are more than approximately 400,000 survivors of childhood and adolescent cancer (diagnosed at ages 0 to 19 years) alive in the United States. The number of survivors will continue to increase, given that the incidence of childhood cancer has been rising slightly in recent decades and that survival rates overall are improving.

The overall outlook for children with cancer has improved greatly over the last half-century. In 1975, just over 50 percent of children diagnosed with cancer before age 20 years survived at least 5 years. In 2004-2010, more than 80 percent of children diagnosed with cancer before age 20 years survived at least 5 years.

Although survival rates for most childhood cancers have improved in recent decades, the improvement has been especially dramatic for a few cancers, particularly acute lymphoblastic leukemia, which is the most common childhood cancer. Improved treatments introduced beginning in the 1970s raised the 5-year survival rate for childhood acute lymphoblastic leukemia from less than 10 percent in the 1960s to about 90 percent in 2003-2009. Survival rates for childhood non-Hodgkin lymphoma have also increased dramatically, from less than 50 percent in the late 1970s to 85 percent in 2003-2009.

By contrast, survival rates remain very low for some cancer types, for some age groups, and for some cancers within a site. For example, median survival for children with diffuse intrinsic pontine glioma (a type of brain tumor) is less than 1 year from diagnosis. Among children with Wilms tumor (a type of kidney cancer), older children (those diagnosed between ages 10 and 16 years) have worse 5-year survival rates than younger children. For soft tissue sarcomas, 5-year survival rates among children and adolescents ages 0 to 19 years range from 64 percent (rhabdomyosarcoma) to 72 percent (Ewing sarcoma). And 5-year survival rates for central nervous system cancers range from 70 percent (medulloblastoma) to 85 percent (astrocytoma).

The cancer mortality rate—the number of deaths due to cancer per 100,000 people per year—among children ages 0 to 19 years declined by more than 50 percent from 1975-1977 to 2007-2010. More specifically, the mortality rate was slightly more than 5 per 100,000 children in 1975 and about 2.3 per 100,000 children in 2010. However, despite the overall decrease in mortality, nearly 2,000 children die of cancer each year in the United States, indicating that new advances and continued research to identify effective treatments are required to further reduce childhood cancer mortality.

Possible Causes of Cancer in Children

The causes of most childhood cancers are not known. About 5 percent of all cancers in children are caused by an inherited mutation (a genetic mutation that can be passed from parents to their children). For example, 25 to 30 percent of cases of retinoblastoma, a cancer of the eye that develops mainly in children, are caused by an inherited mutation in a gene called RB1. However, retinoblastoma accounts for only about 3 percent of all cancers in children.   Inherited mutations associated with certain familial syndromes, such as Li-Fraumeni syndrome, Beckwith-Wiedemann syndrome, Fanconi anemia syndrome, Noonan syndrome, and von Hippel-Lindau syndrome, also increase the risk of childhood cancer.

Genetic mutations that cause cancer can also arise during the development of a fetus in the womb. For example, one in every 100 children is born with a genetic abnormality that increases risk for leukemia, although only one child in 8,000 with that abnormality actually develops leukemia.

Children who have Down syndrome, a genetic condition caused by the presence of an extra copy of chromosome 21, are 10 to 20 times more likely to develop leukemia than children without Down syndrome. However, only a very small proportion of childhood leukemia is linked to Down syndrome.

Most cancers in children, like those in adults, are thought to develop as a result of mutations in genes that lead to uncontrolled cell growth and eventually cancer. In adults, these gene mutations are often the result of exposure to environmental factors, such as cigarette smoke, asbestos, and ultraviolet radiation from the sun. However, environmental causes of childhood cancer have been difficult to identify, partly because cancer in children is rare, and partly because it is difficult to determine what children might have been exposed to early in their development.

Many studies have shown that exposure to ionizing radiation can damage DNA, which can lead to the development of childhood leukemia and possibly other cancers. For example, children and adolescents who were exposed to radiation from the World War II atomic bomb blasts had an elevated risk of leukemia, and children and adults who were exposed to radiation from accidents at nuclear power plants had an elevated risk for thyroid cancer. Children whose mothers had x-rays during pregnancy (that is, children who were exposed before birth) and children who were exposed after birth to diagnostic medical radiation from computed tomography scans also have an increased risk of some cancers.

Studies of other possible environmental risk factors, including parental exposure to cancer-causing chemicals, prenatal exposure to pesticides, childhood exposure to common infectious agents, and living near a nuclear power plant, have so far produced mixed results. Whereas some studies have found associations between these factors and risk of some cancers in children, other studies have found no such associations. Higher risks of cancer have not been seen in children of patients treated for sporadic cancer (cancer not caused by an inherited mutation).

Cancer occurs more frequently in adolescents and young adults ages 15 to 39 years than in younger children, although incidence in this group is still much lower than in older adults. According to NCI's Surveillance, Epidemiology, and End Results (SEER) program, each year in 2001-2007 there were:

- 32.1 cancer diagnoses per 100,000 children ages 0 to 14 years
- 138.6 cancer diagnoses per 100,000 adolescents and young adults ages 15 to 39 years
- 2,053.8 cancer diagnoses per 100,000 people aged 40 years or older

About 70,000 adolescents and young adults ages 15 to 39 years are diagnosed with cancer in the United States each year.

Adolescents and young adults are often diagnosed with different types of cancer than either younger children or older adults. For example, adolescents and young adults are more likely than either younger children or older adults to be diagnosed with Hodgkin lymphoma, melanoma, testicular cancer, thyroid cancer, and sarcoma. However, the incidence of specific cancer types varies widely across the adolescent and young adult age continuum.

The 5-year overall survival rate among adolescents ages 15 to 19 years with cancer exceeded 80 percent in 2003-2007, similar to that among younger children. However, for specific diagnoses, survival is lower for 15- to 19-year-olds than for younger children. For example, the 5-year survival rate for acute lymphoblastic leukemia in 2003-2007 was 91 percent for children younger than 15 years compared with 78 percent for adolescent ages 15 to 19 years.

Some evidence suggests that adolescents and young adults with acute lymphoblastic leukemia may have better outcomes if they are treated with pediatric treatment regimens than if they receive adult treatment regimens. The improvement in 5-year survival rates for 15- to 19-year-olds with acute lymphoblastic leukemia—from approximately 50 percent in the early 1990s to 78 percent in 2003-2007—may reflect greater use of these pediatric treatment regimens. In 2000-2010, mortality rates for 15- to 19-year-olds declined at a slightly faster rate than those for younger children (by 2.6 percent per year versus 1.8 percent per year).

Treatment

Children who have cancer are often treated at a children's cancer center, which is a hospital or a unit within a hospital that specializes in diagnosing and treating children and adolescents who have cancer. Most children's cancer centers treat patients up to 20 years of age. The health professionals at these centers have specific training and expertise to provide comprehensive care for children, adolescents, and their families.

Children's cancer centers also participate in clinical trials. The improvements in survival for children with cancer that have occurred over the past half century have been achieved because of treatment advances that were studied and proven to be effective in clinical trials.

More than 90 percent of children and adolescents who are diagnosed with cancer each year in the United States are cared for at a children's cancer center that is affiliated with the NCI-supported Children's Oncology Group (COG). COG is the world's largest organization that performs clinical research to improve the care and treatment of children and adolescents with cancer. Each year, approximately 4,000 children who are diagnosed with cancer enroll in a COG-sponsored clinical trial.

Every children's cancer center that participates in COG has met strict standards of excellence for childhood cancer care. Families can ask their pediatrician or family doctor for a referral to a children's cancer center. Families and health professionals can call NCI's Cancer Information Service (CIS) at 1–800–4–CANCER to learn more about children's cancer centers that belong to COG.

After Treatment

Survivors of childhood cancer need follow-up care and enhanced medical surveillance for the rest of their lives because of the risk of complications that can occur many years after they complete treatment for their cancer. Health problems that develop months or years after treatment has ended are known as late effects. Indeed, long-term follow-up analysis of a cohort of survivors of childhood cancer treated between 1970 and 1986 has shown that cancer survivors remain at risk of complications and premature death as they age, with more than half of survivors having experienced a severe or disabling complication or even death by the time they reach age 50 years. It is not known whether children treated in more recent periods will experience similar risks of late complications.

The specific late effects that a person who was treated for childhood cancer might experience depend on the type and location of his or her cancer, the type of treatment he or she received, and patient-related factors, such as age at diagnosis.

Children who were treated for bone cancer, brain tumors, and Hodgkin lymphoma, or who received radiation to their chest, abdomen, or pelvis, have the highest risk of serious late effects from their cancer treatment, including second cancers, joint replacement, hearing loss, and congestive heart failure.

It's important for childhood cancer survivors to have regular medical follow-up examinations so any health problems that occur can be identified and treated as soon as possible. It is also important to keep a record of the cancer treatment that someone received as a child. This record should include:

- The type and stage of cancer
- Date of diagnosis and dates of any relapses
- Types and dates of imaging tests
- Contact information for the hospitals and doctors who provided treatment
- Names and total doses of all chemotherapy drugs used in treatment

- The parts of the body that were treated with radiation and the total doses of radiation that were given
- Types and dates of all surgeries
- Any other cancer treatments received
- Any serious complications that occurred during treatment and how those complications were treated
- The date that cancer treatment was completed

Several cancer support organizations have developed kits that can help parents keep track of this information. The record should be kept in a safe place, and copies of the record should be given to all doctors or other health care providers who are involved with the child's follow-up care, even as the child grows into adulthood. Many children's cancer centers have follow-up clinics where survivors of childhood cancer can go for follow-up until they reach their early 20s. Some cancer centers are now creating clinics dedicated to follow-up care for long-term cancer survivors.

CARING FOR THE CAREGIVER

Giving care can mean helping with daily needs. These include going to doctor visits, making meals, and picking up medicines. It can also mean helping your loved one cope with feelings. Like when he or she feels sad or angry. Sometimes having someone to talk to is what your loved one needs most.

While giving care, it's normal to put your own needs and feelings aside. But putting your needs aside for a long time is not good for your health. You need to take care of yourself, too. If you don't, you may not be able to care for others. This is why you need to take good care of you.

It's common to feel stressed and overwhelmed at this time. Like your loved one, you may feel angry, sad, or worried. Try to share your feelings with others who can help you. It can help to talk about how you feel. You could even talk to a counselor or social worker.

Understanding your feelings

You probably have many feelings as you take care of your loved one. There is no right way for you to feel. Each person is different. The first step to understanding your feelings is to know that they're normal. Give yourself some time to think through them. Some feelings that may come and go are:

- Sadness. It's okay to feel sad. But if it lasts for more than 2 weeks, and it keeps you from doing what you need to do, you may be depressed.
- Anger. You may be angry at yourself or family members. You may be angry at the person you're caring for. Or you may be angry that your loved one has cancer. Sometimes anger comes from fear, panic, or stress. If you are angry, try to think of what makes you feel this way. Knowing the cause may help.
- Grief. You may be feeling a loss of what you value most. This may be your loved one's health. Or it may be the loss of the day-to-day life you had before the cancer was found. Let yourself grieve these losses.
- Guilt. Feeling guilty is common, too. You may think you aren't helping enough. Or you may feel guilty that you are healthy.
- Loneliness. You can feel lonely, even with lots of people around you. You may feel that no one understands your problems. You may also be spending less time with others.

What may help

Talk with someone if your feelings get in the way of daily life. Maybe you have a family member, friend, priest, pastor, or spiritual leader to talk to. Your doctor may also be able to help.

Here are some other things that may help you:

- Know that we all make mistakes whenever we have a lot on our minds. No one is perfect.
- Cry or express your feelings. You don't have to pretend to be cheerful. It's okay to show that you are sad or upset.
- Focus on things that are worth your time and energy. Let small things go for now. For example, don't fold clothes if you are tired.
- Remind yourself that you are doing the best you can.
- Spend time alone to think about your feelings.

Many people who were once caregivers say they did too much on their own. Some wished that they had asked for help sooner. Be honest about what you can do. Think about tasks you can give to others. And let go of tasks that aren't so important at this time. Asking for help also helps your loved one.

Don't be afraid to ask for help. Remember, if you get help for yourself:

- You may stay healthier and have more energy.
- Your loved one may feel less guilty about your help.
- Other helpers may offer time and skills that you don't have.

How can others help you?

People may want to help you but don't know what you need. Here are some things you can ask them to do:

- Help with tasks such as cooking, cleaning and shopping
- Talk with you and share your feelings.
- Help with driving errands such as doctor visits and picking up your children
- Find information you need.
- Tell others how your loved one is doing.

Know that some people may say, "No."

Some people may not be able to help. There could be one or more reasons such as:

- They may be coping with their own problems.
- They may not have time right now.
- They may not know how to help.
- They may feel uneasy around people who are sick.

Making time for yourself

Taking time for yourself can help you be a better caregiver. That's even truer if you have health problems. You may want to:

- Find nice things you can do for yourself. Even just a few minutes can help. You could watch TV, call a friend, work on a hobby, or do anything that you enjoy.
- Be active. Even light exercise such as walking, stretching, or dancing can make you less tired. Yard work, playing with kids or pets, or working in the garden are helpful, too.
- Find ways to connect with friends. Are there places you can meet others who are close to you? Or can you chat or get support by phone or email?
- Give yourself more time off. Ask friends or family members to pitch in. Take time to rest.

Do something for yourself each day. It doesn't matter how small it is. Whatever you do, don't neglect yourself.

Caring for your body

You may feel too busy to think about your own health. But taking care of your body gives you strength. Then you can take care of someone else. Keep up with your own health needs. Try to:

- Go to all your checkups

- Take your medicines
- Eat healthy meals
- Get enough rest
- Exercise
- Make time to relax

Did you have health problems before you became a caregiver? If so, now it's even more important to take care of yourself. Also, adding extra stressors to your life can cause new health problems. Be sure to tell your doctor if you notice any new changes in your body.

Finding meaning during cancer

Cancer causes many caregivers to look at life in new ways. They think about the purpose of life. And they often focus on what they value most. You and your loved one may question why cancer has come into your lives. You may long for things to be like they were before the disease. But you may also see good things that come out of it, such as it bringing you closer. It's normal to see illness in both good and bad ways.

Cancer can affect one's faith in different ways. Some people turn toward their beliefs. Others turn away from them. It is common to question your faith during this time. For some, looking for meaning is a way to cope. Some ways to find meaning are:

- Read or listen to uplifting materials.
- Pray or meditate.
- Talk with a priest, pastor, or spiritual leader.
- Go to religious or spiritual services.
- Talk to other caregivers.
- Look at books or brochures for people dealing with cancer. Ask for them at your place of worship. Also, check at libraries for these materials.

Going With Your Loved One to Medical Visits

Your loved one may ask you to come to doctor visits. This may be a key role for you. Here are some tips for going to the doctor:

- Know how to get there. Give yourself enough time.
- Write down questions you need to ask. Also write down things you want to tell the doctor.

- Keep a folder of your loved one's health information. Bring this folder to each visit.
- Bring all the medicine bottles with you, or keep a list of the names and doses. Bring this list to each visit.

Talking with the health care provider

Sometimes, people have trouble with medical visits. They don't understand what the doctor says. Or they forget things. Here are some tips for talking with the health care provider:
- If you don't understand an answer, ask the question in a different way.
- If you need to know more, ask.
- Let your doctor or nurse know what your worries are.
- Before you leave the visit, make sure you know what the next steps are for your loved one's care.
- Take notes. Or ask if you can tape-record the visit.
- Let the doctor know if your loved one has had changes or new symptoms.

Questions to ask the doctor or health care team
- What health records should we bring?
- How can we prepare for treatment?
- How long will the treatment take?
- Can he or she go to and from treatment alone?
- How can I help my loved one feel better during treatment?
- Can I be there during treatment?
- What are the side effects of the treatment?
- After treatment, what do we need to watch for? When should we call you?
- How do we file for insurance? Who can help us with insurance?

Asking about pain

Many caregivers say that they are afraid to ask about pain. They worry that it means the cancer is getting worse. Or some think that pain is normal, and their loved one just has to accept it. This is not true. People who have their pain managed can focus on healing. They can enjoy life more.

The doctor should continue to ask about pain and other side effects. But it's up to you and your loved one to be sure that the doctor knows about any pain your loved one feels. Pain can be managed during treatment. The key is to talk about pain and other symptoms at each visit. Your loved one does not have to suffer.

Don't be afraid to ask for stronger pain medicine. Sometimes larger doses help. These drugs rarely cause people with cancer to get addicted. Instead, they can help your loved one feel better. He or she will be able to focus on day-to-day things instead of being in pain.

Talking With Others

Nearly all caregivers and their partners feel more stress than usual in their relationship. They must deal with many decisions and changes. Some couples find that their bonds get stronger during cancer treatment. Others find they get weaker. Try to be open about your stress and its causes. You may want to:

Talk about how each of you feels:
- Share how you are each coping.
- Look at things that are causing you both stress.
- Talk about choices you can make together.
- Try to be grateful for each other.

Make time to focus on things besides cancer.

Talk with your partner if you find that your sex life is different than it used to be. There can be many causes:
- You or your partner is tired.
- Your relationship feels strained.
- If your partner is the patient: Either of you may not feel good about how your partner looks.
- You may be afraid you will hurt your partner.
- The treatment might be affecting your partner's ability to perform. He or she may be in pain or depressed.

You can still be close as a couple in spite of these issues. Staying close is also about sharing feelings and understanding. You can:
- Talk about closeness and your sex life.
- Talk about your hopes for the future.
- Try not to judge each other.
- Protect your time together.
- Be patient and take things slowly.
- Talk to a counselor or your support group.

Other family members and friends

Did your family have problems before cancer? These problems are likely to be more intense now. This is true if you are caring for a spouse, child, or parent. Your new role as a caregiver may cause feelings you didn't expect.

Talk with the people close to you. Try to be open and caring. Ask a counselor to hold a family meeting if needed. During stressful times, ask someone else to update others about how your loved one is doing.

Dealing with help you don't need

Sometimes people offer help you don't need. Thank them for their concern. Tell them you'll let them know if you need anything.

Some people may offer unwanted advice. They may do this because they don't know what else to say. It's up to you to decide how to deal with this. You don't have to respond at all. Otherwise, thank them and let it go. Tell them you are taking steps to help your family.

Your kids

Children start to understand the world around them at a very young age. It is important to be honest with them. They need to know the truth about your loved one. Otherwise, they will think the worst. Let them know how you feel, too. Some tips for talking with kids:

- Tell them about cancer. Let them know that there is nothing they did to cause cancer. And they can't catch it from someone else.
- Let them know their feelings are okay. Tell them you understand if they are upset, angry, sad, or scared. Remind them that no matter what happens, you will always love them.
- Tell them the truth with love and hope. Let them know that your loved one is getting good care and that you hope he or she will get well again. But don't try to promise them a good outcome if you aren't sure of one.
- Listen to them. Ask them how they feel and what they are worried about. If they're young, ask them to draw a picture or play with dolls to show you how they feel
- Stay involved. You may be with your loved one who is sick more often right now. Try to spend time with your kids in any way you can. Take them to the store with you or eat meals with them. Ask them about their day. Leave them notes or call them when you can.

Remember

As a caregiver, try to remember to:
- Strike a balance each day.
- Focus on your needs, too.
- Care for yourself while caring for your loved one.
- Make time for resting and relaxing.

Life-changing events often give people the chance to grow. They may help people see what's most important to them. Many say that caring for someone with cancer changed them forever. They used their strengths to support their loved one. And they learned more about themselves along the way.

4

Diabetes

Over 29.1 million Americans (9.3% of the population) have diabetes, making it a leading cause of heart attacks, strokes, blindness, kidney failure, limb amputation, as well as the seventh leading cause of death. Over 8 million of these have diabetes or are prediabetic and do not know.

In 2009-2012, based on fasting glucose or A1C levels, 37% of U.S. adults aged 20 years or older had prediabetes (51% of those aged 65 years or older). Applying this percentage to the entire U.S. population in 2012 yields an estimated 86 million Americans aged 20 years or older with prediabetes.

On the basis of fasting glucose or A1C levels, and after adjusting for population age differences, the percentage of U.S. adults aged 20 years or older with prediabetes in 2009-2012 was similar for nonHispanic whites (35%), non-Hispanic blacks (39%), and Hispanics (38%).

The total direct and indirect cost of diabetes in the U.S. is $245 billion with direct medical costs amounting to $176 billion and $69 billion from disability, work loss and premature death.

WHAT IS DIABETES?

Diabetes is a group of diseases marked by high levels of blood glucose resulting from problems in how insulin is produced, how insulin works, or both. People with diabetes may develop serious complications such as heart disease, stroke, kidney failure, blindness, and premature death.

Type 1 Diabetes

Type 1 diabetes was previously called insulin-dependent diabetes mellitus or juvenile-onset diabetes. Although disease onset can occur at any age, the peak age for diagnosis is in the mid-teens. Type 1 diabetes develops when the cells that produce the hormone insulin, known as the beta cells, in the pancreas are destroyed. This destruction is initiated or mediated by the body's immune system and limits or completely eliminates the production and secretion of insulin, the hormone that is required to lower blood glucose levels. To survive, people with type 1 diabetes must have insulin delivered by injection or a pump. In adults, type 1 diabetes accounts for approximately 5% of all diagnosed cases of diabetes. There is no known way to prevent type 1 diabetes. Several clinical trials for preventing type 1 diabetes are currently in progress with additional studies being planned.

Type 2 Diabetes

Type 2 diabetes was previously called non–insulin-dependent diabetes mellitus or adult-onset diabetes because the peak age of onset is usually later than type 1 diabetes. In adults, type 2 diabetes accounts for about 90% to 95% of all diagnosed cases of diabetes. Type 2 diabetes usually begins with insulin resistance, a disorder in which the cells primarily within the muscles, liver, and fat tissue do not use insulin properly. As the need for insulin rises, the beta cells in the pancreas gradually lose the ability to produce sufficient quantities of the hormone. The role of insulin resistance as opposed to beta cell dysfunction differs among individuals, with some having primarily insulin resistance and only a minor defect in insulin secretion, and others with slight insulin resistance and primarily a lack of insulin secretion. The risk for developing type 2 diabetes is associated with older age, obesity, family history of diabetes, and history of gestational diabetes, impaired glucose metabolism, physical inactivity, and race/ethnicity. African Americans, Hispanics/Latinos, American Indians, some Asians, and Native Hawaiians or other Pacific Islanders are at particularly high risk for type 2 diabetes and its complications. Type 2 diabetes in children and adolescents, although uncommon, is being diagnosed more frequently among American Indians, African Americans, Hispanics/Latinos, Asians, and Pacific Islanders.

Gestational diabetes

Gestational diabetes is a form of glucose intolerance diagnosed during the second or third trimester of pregnancy. During pregnancy, increasing blood glucose levels increase the risk for both mother and fetus and require treatment to reduce problems for the mother and infant. Treatment may include diet, regular physical activity, or insulin. Shortly after pregnancy, 5% to 10% of women with gestational diabetes continue to have high blood glucose levels and are diagnosed as having diabetes, usually type 2. The risk factors for gestational diabetes are similar to those for type 2 diabetes. The occurrence of gestational diabetes itself is a risk factor for developing recurrent gestational diabetes with future pregnancies and subsequent development of type 2 diabetes. Also, the children of women who had gestational diabetes during pregnancies may be at risk of developing obesity and diabetes. Other types of diabetes such as maturity-onset diabetes of youth or latent autoimmune diabetes in adults, among others, are caused by specific genetic conditions or from surgery, medications, infections, pancreatic disease, or other illnesses. Such types of diabetes account for 1% to 5% of all diagnosed cases.

WHAT IS PREDIABETES?

Prediabetes is a condition in which individuals have high blood glucose or hemoglobin A1C levels but not high enough to be classified as diabetes. People with prediabetes have an increased risk of developing type 2 diabetes, heart disease, and stroke, but not everyone with prediabetes will progress to diabetes. The Diabetes Prevention Program, a large prevention study of people at high risk for diabetes, showed that lifestyle intervention that resulted in weight loss and increased physical activity in this population can prevent or delay type 2 diabetes and in some cases return blood glucose levels to within the normal range. Other international studies have shown similar results.

Most people with prediabetes don't have any symptoms. Your doctor can test your blood to find out if your blood glucose levels are higher than normal. If you are 45 years old or older, your doctor may recommend that you be tested for prediabetes, especially if you are overweight. Being overweight is a key contributor, along with inactivity, to prediabetes. If your body mass index (BMI) is higher than 25, you are overweight. BMI is a measure of your weight relative to your height. If you're not sure if you are overweight, ask your doctor.

Even if you are younger than 45, consider getting tested for prediabetes if you are overweight and

- are physically inactive
- have a parent, brother, or sister with diabetes
- have high blood pressure or high cholesterol—blood fat
- have abnormal levels of HDL, or good, cholesterol or triglycerides— another type of blood fat
- had gestational diabetes—diabetes that develops only during pregnancy—or gave birth to a baby weighing more than 9 pounds
- are African American, Alaska Native, American Indian, Asian American, Hispanic/Latino, or Pacific Islander American
- have polycystic ovary syndrome, also called PCOS
- have a dark, velvety rash around your neck or armpits
- have blood vessel problems affecting your heart, brain, or legs

If your test results are normal, you should be retested in 3 years. If you have prediabetes, ask your doctor if you should be tested again in 1 year.

What Can I Do About Prediabetes?

Losing weight—at least 5 to 10 percent of your starting weight—can prevent or delay diabetes or even reverse prediabetes. That's 10 to 20 pounds for someone who weighs 200 pounds. You can lose weight by cutting the amount of calories and fat you consume and by being physically active at least 30 to 60 minutes every day. Physical activity also helps your body use the hormone insulin properly. Your body needs insulin to use glucose for energy.

Medicine can help control the amount of glucose in your blood. Ask your doctor if medicine to control glucose is right for you.

The National Diabetes Education Program's Small Steps. Big Rewards. Prevent Type 2 Diabetes campaign has more information about preventing diabetes at www.ndep.nih.gov.

The signs and symptoms of diabetes are

- being very thirsty
- urinating often
- feeling very hungry

- feeling very tired
- losing weight without trying
- sores that heal slowly
- dry, itchy skin
- feelings of pins and needles in your feet
- losing feeling in your feet
- blurry eyesight

Some people with diabetes don't have any of these signs or symptoms. The only way to know if you have diabetes is to have your doctor do a blood test.

You may have diabetes problems if:

- your blood pressure is 140 over 80, written as 140/80, or higher
- you have pain in your chest
- you have blurry or double vision, or feel pain or pressure in your eyes
- you have foot problems—such as blisters, ingrown toenails, or cracked skin—that get infected
- your arms, hands, legs, or feet feel numb, or you feel shooting pains

Some diabetes problems don't have symptoms at first. For example, you cannot tell if your kidneys are damaged until they stop working altogether. Your doctor should test your urine every year to see how well your kidneys are working.

Controlling your blood glucose, blood pressure, and cholesterol can make a big difference in staying healthy. Talk with your doctor about what your ABC goals should be and how to reach them. A stands for the A1C test—a measure of what your blood glucose has been for the last three months. B is for blood pressure, and C is for cholesterol.

You can take these steps each day to reach your ABC goals:

- Follow the healthy eating plan that you and your doctor or dietitian have discussed.
- Be physically active for 30 to 60 minutes most days.
- Take your medicines as directed and keep taking them, even after you've reached your goals.
- If you smoke, quit.
- Ask your doctor if you should take aspirin to prevent a heart attack or stroke.
- Check your feet every day for cuts, blisters, sores, swelling, redness, or sore toenails.

Diabetes causes abnormally high blood glucose levels, either because the body does not produce insulin (Type 1) or the body does not produce enough insulin to function properly (Type 2). A third type, gestational diabetes, affects females during pregnancy. While Type 1 diabetes is primarily genetic, Type 2 diabetes (usually closely related to obesity), can be prevented through proper diet and exercise. Type 2 diabetes can cause kidney damage, heart disease and blindness. It is also a leading cause of death in both men and women. Lose extra weight, exercise and eat a healthy diet to prevent diabetes.

Public health officials are working on diabetes prevention campaigns which promote healthier diets and active lifestyles.

Diabetes can be treated and managed by healthful eating, regular physical activity, and medications to lower blood glucose levels. Another critical part of diabetes management is reducing cardiovascular disease risk factors, such as high blood pressure, high lipid levels, and tobacco use. Patient education and self-care practices also are important aspects of disease management that help people with diabetes stay healthy.

- People with type 1 diabetes must have insulin delivered by injection or a pump to survive.
- Many people with type 2 diabetes can control their blood glucose by following a healthy meal plan and a program of regular physical activity, losing excess weight, and taking medications. Medications for each individual with diabetes will often change during the course of the disease. Insulin also is commonly used to control blood glucose in people with type 2 diabetes.
- Blood glucose control reduces the risk of developing the eye, nerve, and kidney complications of diabetes.
- Hypoglycemia or low blood glucose is a complication of diabetes treatment with insulin or certain oral medications that can have serious consequences such as seizures, unconsciousness, or death. Older patients with type 2 diabetes and children with type 1 diabetes are at particularly high risk for adverse outcomes associated with hypoglycemia.
- Individual blood glucose targets, with the selection of targets based on the potential risks and benefits to the patient, are encouraged for people with diabetes.
- Self-management education or training focuses on self-care behaviors, such as healthy eating, being active, adhering to medications, learning coping skills, and monitoring blood glucose.

- Many people with diabetes also need to take medications to control their blood pressure and to control their cholesterol.

COMPLICATIONS

Diabetes can affect many parts of the body and is associated with serious complications, such as heart disease and stroke, blindness, kidney failure, and lower-limb amputation. Some complications, especially microvascular (e.g., eye, kidney, and nerve) disease, can be reduced with good glucose control. Also, early detection and treatment of complications can prevent progression, so monitoring with dilated eye exams, urine tests, and foot exams is essential. Because the risk of cardiovascular disease is increased in diabetes and prediabetes, blood pressure and lipid management, along with smoking cessation, are especially important. By working together, people with diagnosed diabetes, their support network, and their health care providers can reduce the occurrence of these and other complications. Figures quoted are the latest available.

Hypoglycemia and Hyperglycemic Crisis

Hypoglycemia

- In 2011, about 282,000 emergency room visits for adults aged 18 years or older had hypoglycemia as the first-listed diagnosis and diabetes as another diagnosis

Hyperglycemic crisis

- In 2011, about 175,000 emergency room visits for people of all ages had hyperglycemic crisis, e.g., diabetic ketoacidosis and hyperglycemic hyperosmolar state, as the first-listed diagnosis.
- In 2010, among adults aged 20 years or older, hyperglycemic crisis caused 2,361 deaths.

High Blood Pressure

• In 2009–2012, of adults aged 18 years or older with diagnosed diabetes, 71% had blood pressure greater than or equal to 140/90 millimeters of mercury or used prescription medications to lower high blood pressure.

High Blood LDL Cholesterol

• In 2009–2012, of adults aged 18 years or older with diagnosed diabetes, 65% had blood LDL cholesterol greater than or equal to 100 mg/dl or used cholesterol-lowering medications.

Heart Disease and Stroke

• In 2003–2006, after adjusting for population age differences, cardiovascular disease death rates were about 1.7 times higher among adults aged 18 years or older with diagnosed diabetes than among adults without diagnosed diabetes.
• In 2010, after adjusting for population age differences, hospitalization rates for heart attack were 1.8 times higher among adults aged 20 years or older with diagnosed diabetes than among adults without diagnosed diabetes.
• In 2010, after adjusting for population age differences, hospitalization rates for stroke were 1.5 times higher among adults with diagnosed diabetes aged 20 years or older compared to those without diagnosed diabetes.

Blindness and Eye Problems

• In 2005–2008, of adults with diabetes aged 40 years or older, 4.2 million (28.5%) people had diabetic retinopathy, damage to the small blood vessels in the retina that may result in loss of vision.
• In 2005–2008, of adults with diabetes aged 40 years or older, 655,000 (4.4%) had advanced diabetic retinopathy—with conditions such as

clinically significant macular edema and proliferative diabetic retinopathy—that could lead to severe vision loss.

Kidney Disease

- Diabetes was listed as the primary cause of kidney failure in 44% of all new cases in 2011.
- In 2011, 49,677 people of all ages began treatment for kidney failure due to diabetes.
- In 2011, a total of 228,924 people of all ages with kidney failure due to diabetes were living on chronic dialysis or with a kidney transplant.

Amputations

- In 2010, about 73,000 non-traumatic lower-limb amputations were performed in adults aged 20 years or older with diagnosed diabetes.
- About 60% of non-traumatic lower-limb amputations among people aged 20 years or older occur in people with diagnosed diabetes.

Other Conditions and Complications

- People with diabetes may have or develop other complications or conditions, such as nerve disease, nonalcoholic fatty liver disease, periodontal (gum) disease, hearing loss, erectile dysfunction, depression, and complications of pregnancy, among others.

WHY DO YOU NEED TO TAKE CARE OF YOUR DIABETES?

Over time, diabetes can lead to serious problems with your blood vessels, heart, nerves, kidneys, mouth, eyes, and feet. These problems can lead to an amputation, which is surgery to remove a damaged toe, foot, or leg, for example.

The most serious problem caused by diabetes is heart disease. When you have diabetes, you are more than twice as likely as people without diabetes to have heart disease or a stroke. With diabetes, you may not have the usual signs or symptoms of a heart attack. The best way to take care of your health is to work with your health care team to keep your blood glucose, blood pressure, and cholesterol levels in your target range. Targets are numbers you aim for.

Your Health Care Team

Most people with diabetes get care from primary care providers, such as internists, family physicians, or pediatricians. A team of health care providers can also improve your diabetes care. In addition to a primary care provider, your health care team may include

- an endocrinologist for more specialized diabetes care
- a dietitian, a nurse, or a certified diabetes educator—experts who can provide information about managing diabetes
- a counselor or mental health professional
- a pharmacist
- a dentist
- an ophthalmologist or an optometrist for eye care
- a podiatrist for foot care

If diabetes makes you feel sad or angry, or if you have other problems that worry you, you should talk with a counselor or mental health professional. Your doctor or certified diabetes educator can help you find a counselor. Talk with your doctor about what vaccines and immunizations, or shots, you should get to keep from getting sick. Preventing illness is an important part of taking care of your diabetes.

When you see members of your health care team, ask lots of questions. Prepare a list of questions before your visit. Be sure you understand everything you need to know about taking care of your diabetes.

5

Kidney Disease

Almost 4 million people in the U.S. have been diagnosed with kidney disease which is the ninth-leading cause of death for both male and female, according to the Centers for Disease Control and Prevention.

The kidneys are two bean-shaped organs, each about the size of a fist. They are located just below the rib cage, one on each side of the spine. Every day, the two kidneys filter about 120 to 150 quarts of blood to produce about 1 to 2 quarts of urine, composed of wastes and extra fluid. Children produce less urine than adults and the amount produced depends on their age. The kidneys work around the clock; a person does not control what they do. Ureters are the thin tubes of muscle—one on each side of the bladder—that carry urine from each of the kidneys to the bladder. The bladder stores urine until the person finds an appropriate time and place to urinate.

Every day, the two kidneys filter about 120 to 150 quarts of blood to produce about 1 to 2 quarts of urine, composed of wastes and extra fluid.

The kidney is not one large filter. Each kidney is made up of about a million filtering units called nephrons. Each nephron filters a small amount of blood. The nephron includes a filter, called a glomerulus, and a tubule. The nephrons work through a two-step process. The glomerulus lets fluid and waste products pass through it; however, it prevents blood cells and large molecules, mostly proteins, from passing. The filtered fluid then passes through the tubule, which changes the fluid by sending needed minerals back to the bloodstream and removing wastes. The final product becomes urine.

The kidneys also control the level of minerals such as sodium, phosphorus, and potassium in the body, and produce an important hormone to prevent anemia. Anemia is a condition in which the number of red blood cells is less than normal, resulting in less oxygen carried to the body's cells.

WHAT THE KIDNEYS DO

The kidneys are important because they keep the composition, or makeup, of the blood stable, which lets the body function. They
- prevent the buildup of wastes and extra fluid in the body
- keep levels of electrolytes stable, such as sodium, potassium, and phosphate
- make hormones that help
- regulate blood pressure
- make red blood cells
- bones stay strong

KIDNEY DISEASE

Kidney disease means that the kidneys are damaged and can't filter blood like they should. This damage can cause wastes to build up in the body. It can also cause other problems that can harm your health.

For most people, kidney damage occurs slowly over many years, often due to diabetes or high blood pressure. This is called chronic kidney disease. When someone has a sudden change in kidney function—because of illness, injury, or have taken certain medications—this is called acute kidney injury. This can occur in a person with normal kidneys or in someone who already has kidney problems.

People with kidney disease often have high blood pressure, and are more likely to have a stroke or heart attack. They can also develop anemia (low number of red blood cells), bone disease, and malnutrition. Kidney disease can get worse over time, and may lead to kidney failure.

Diabetes and high blood pressure are the most common causes of kidney disease. Other important causes include glomerulonephritis and polycystic kidney disease. Your provider will want to know why you have kidney disease so your treatment can also address the cause.

Treatment may help slow kidney disease and keep the kidneys healthier longer. Medicines and diet and lifestyle changes are important for people with kidney disease.

Take these steps to help keep your kidneys healthier longer:

Choose foods with less salt (sodium).

Keep your blood pressure at or below the target set by your health care provider. For most people, the blood pressure target is less than 140/90 mm Hg.

Keep your blood glucose in the target range, if you have diabetes.

Work with your health care team to figure out the treatment plan that makes the most sense for you. With proper management, you may never need dialysis or, at least, not for a very long time.

KIDNEY FAILURE

Your kidneys filter wastes from your blood and regulate other functions of your body. When your kidneys fail, you need treatment to replace the work your kidneys normally perform.

Developing kidney failure means you have some decisions to make about your treatment. You may choose to forgo treatment. If you choose to receive treatment, your choices include hemodialysis, which requires a machine used to filter your blood outside your body; peritoneal dialysis, which uses the lining of your belly to filter your blood inside the body; and kidney transplantation, in which a new kidney is placed in your body. Each treatment has advantages and disadvantages. Your choice of treatment will have a big impact on your day-to-day lifestyle, such as being able to keep a job if you are working. You are the only one who can decide what means most to you. Reading this information is a good way to learn about your options so you can make an informed choice. And, if you find that your choice is not a good fit for your life, you can change treatments. With the help of your health care team, family, and friends, you can lead a full, active life.

When Your Kidneys Fail

Healthy kidneys clean your blood by removing excess fluid, minerals, and wastes. They also make hormones that keep your bones strong and your blood healthy. When your kidneys fail, harmful wastes build up in your body, your blood pressure may rise, and your body may retain excess fluid and not make enough red blood cells. When this happens, you need treatment to replace the work of your failed kidneys.

TREATMENT CHOICES

Hemodialysis

Hemodialysis cleans and filters your blood using a machine to temporarily rid your body of harmful wastes, extra salt, and extra water. Hemodialysis helps control blood pressure and helps your body keep the proper balance of important chemicals such as potassium, sodium, calcium, and bicarbonate.

Dialysis can replace part of the function of your kidneys. Diet, medications, and fluid limits are often needed as well. Your diet, fluids, and the number of medications you need will depend on which treatment you choose.

Hemodialysis uses a special filter called a dialyzer that functions as an artificial kidney to clean your blood. The dialyzer is a canister connected to the hemodialysis machine.

During treatment, your blood travels through tubes into the dialyzer, which filters out wastes, extra salt, and extra water. Then the cleaned blood flows through another set of tubes back into your body. The hemodialysis machine monitors blood flow and removes wastes from the dialyzer.

Hemodialysis is usually done three times a week. Each treatment lasts from 3 to 5 or more hours. During treatment, you can read, write, sleep, talk, or watch TV.

Arteriovenous fistula. Several months before your first hemodialysis treatment, an access to your bloodstream will need to be created. You may need to stay overnight in the hospital, but many patients have their access created on an outpatient basis. This access provides an efficient way for blood to be carried from your body to the dialyzer and back without causing discomfort. The two main types of access are a fistula and a graft.

- A surgeon makes a fistula by using your own blood vessels; an artery is connected directly to a vein, usually in your forearm. The increased blood flow makes the vein grow larger and stronger so it can be used for repeated needle insertions. This kind of access is the preferred type. It may take several weeks to be ready for use.
- A graft connects an artery to a vein by using a synthetic tube. It doesn't need to develop as a fistula does, so it can be used sooner after placement. But a graft is more likely to have problems with infection and clotting.

If your kidney disease has progressed quickly, you may not have time to get a permanent vascular access before you start hemodialysis treatments. You may need to use a catheter-a small, soft tube inserted into a vein in your neck, chest, or leg near the groin-as a temporary access. Some people use a catheter for long-term access as well. Catheters that will be needed for more than about 3 weeks are designed to be placed under the skin to increase comfort and reduce complications.

Hemodialysis is most often done in a dialysis center by patient care technicians who are supervised by nurses. Medicare pays for three hemodialysis treatments each week. If you choose in-center treatment, you will have a fixed time slot three times per week on Monday-Wednesday-Friday or Tuesday-Thursday-Saturday. If you do not get the time slot you want at first, you can ask to be put on a waiting list for the time slot you prefer. For a special event, you may be able to trade times with someone else. You will want to think about the dialysis schedule if you work or have children to care for. Some centers offer in-center nocturnal dialysis. This treatment is done for a longer period at night, while you sleep at the center. Getting more dialysis means fewer diet and fluid limits, and this treatment leaves your days free for work, child care, hobbies, or other tasks.

You can choose to learn how to do your own hemodialysis treatments at home. When you are the only patient, it is possible to do longer or more frequent dialysis, which comes closer to replacing the steady work healthy kidneys do. Daily home hemodialysis (DHHD) is done 5 to 7 days per week for 2 to 3 hours at a time, and you set the schedule. If your health plan will pay for more than three treatments, you might do the short treatments in the mornings or in the evenings. Nocturnal home hemodialysis (NHHD) is done 3 to 6 nights per week while you sleep. Either DHHD or NHHD will allow a more normal diet and fluids, with fewer blood pressure and other medications. Most programs want people doing hemodialysis at home to have a trained partner in the home while they do treatments. Learning to do home hemodialysis is like learning to drive a car—it takes a few weeks and is scary at first, but then it becomes routine. The dialysis center provides the machine and training, plus 24-hour support if you have a question or problem. New machines for home dialysis are smaller and easier to use than in-center ones.

You have a choice of dialysis centers, and most towns have more than one center to choose from. You can visit a center to see if it has the treatments you want or the time slot you need. Some centers will let you use a laptop or cell phone or have visitors, and others will not. Medicare has a list of all U.S. centers on its Dialysis Facility Compare website (http://www.medicare.gov /DialysisFacilityCompare/search.html) with quality ratings for each. Your health plan may have a list of centers you can use. If you choose in-center treatment, you may want the center to be close to your home to reduce your travel time. If you do a home treatment, once you are trained you only need to visit the center once a month. So, the center can be as far away as you are willing to travel once a month.

Possible Complications

Vascular access problems are the most common reason for hospitalization among people on hemodialysis. Common problems include infection, blockage from clotting, and poor blood flow. These problems can keep your treatments from working. You may need to undergo repeated surgeries in order to get a properly functioning access.

Other problems can be caused by rapid changes in your body's water and chemical balance during treatment. Muscle cramps and hypotension-a sudden drop in blood pressure-are two common side effects. Hypotension can make you feel weak, dizzy, or sick to your stomach.

You'll probably need a few months to adjust to hemodialysis. Side effects can often be treated quickly and easily, so you should always report them to your doctor and dialysis staff. You can avoid many side effects if you follow a proper diet, limit your liquid intake, and take your medicines as directed.

Diet for Hemodialysis

Hemodialysis and a proper diet help reduce the wastes that build up in your blood. A dietitian is available at all dialysis centers to help you plan meals according to your doctor's orders. When choosing foods, remember to

- eat balanced amounts of high-protein foods such as meat, chicken, and fish.
- control the amount of potassium you eat. Potassium is a mineral found in salt substitutes; some fruits, such as bananas and oranges; vegetables; chocolate; and nuts. Too much potassium can be dangerous to your heart.
- limit how much you drink. When your kidneys aren't working, water builds up quickly in your body. Too much liquid makes your tissues swell and can lead to high blood pressure, heart trouble, and cramps and low blood pressure during dialysis.
- avoid salt. Salty foods make you thirsty and make your body hold water.
- limit foods such as milk, cheese, nuts, dried beans, and dark colas. These foods contain large amounts of the mineral phosphorus. Too much phosphorus in your blood causes calcium to be pulled from your bones, which makes them weak and brittle and can cause arthritis. To prevent bone problems, your doctor may give you special medicines, which you must take with meals every day as directed.

Pros and Cons

Each person responds differently to similar situations. What may be a negative factor for one person may be a positive one for another. See a list of the general advantages and disadvantages of in-center and home hemodialysis below.

In-Center Hemodialysis

Pros

- Facilities are widely available.
- Trained professionals are with you at all times.
- You can get to know other patients.
- You don't have to have a partner or keep equipment in your home.

Cons

- Treatments are scheduled by the center and are relatively fixed.
- You must travel to the center for treatment.
- This treatment has the strictest diet and fluid limits of all.
- You will need to take-and pay for-more medications.
- You may have more frequent ups and downs in how you feel from day to day.
- It may take a few hours to feel better after a treatment.

Home Hemodialysis

Pros

- You can do it at the times you choose-but you still must do it as often as your doctor orders
- You don't have to travel to a center.
- You gain a sense of independence and control over your treatment.
- Newer machines require less space.
- You will have fewer ups and downs in how you feel from day to day.
- Home hemodialysis is more work-friendly than in-center treatment.
- Your diet and fluids will be much closer to normal
- You can take along new, portable machines on car trips, in campers, or on airplanes.
- You can spend more time with your loved ones.

Cons

- You must have a partner.
- Helping with treatments may be stressful to your family.
- You and your partner need training.
- You need space for storing the machine and supplies at home.
- You may need to take a leave of absence from work to complete training.
- You will need to learn to put in the dialysis needles.
- Daily and nocturnal home hemodialysis are not yet offered in all locations.

Working With Your Health Care Team

Questions you may want to ask:

- Is hemodialysis the best treatment choice for me? Why?
- If I'm treated at a center, can I go to the center of my choice?
- What should I look for in a dialysis center?
- Will my kidney doctor see me at dialysis?
- What does hemodialysis feel like?
- What is self-care dialysis?
- Is home hemodialysis available in my area? How long does it take to learn? Who will train my partner and me?
- What kind of blood access is best for me?
- As a hemodialysis patient, will I be able to keep working? Can I have treatments at night?
- How much should I exercise?
- Who will be on my health care team? How can these people help me?
- With whom can I talk about finances, sexuality, or family concerns?
- How/where can I talk with other people who have faced this decision?

Peritoneal Dialysis

Peritoneal dialysis is another procedure that removes wastes, chemicals, and extra water from your body. This type of dialysis uses the lining of your abdomen, or belly, to filter your blood. This lining is called the peritoneal membrane and acts as the artificial kidney.

A mixture of minerals and sugar dissolved in water, called dialysis solution, travels through a catheter into your belly. The sugar—called dextrose—draws wastes, chemicals, and extra water from the tiny blood vessels in your peritoneal membrane into the dialysis solution. After several hours, the used solution is drained from your abdomen through the tube, taking the wastes from your blood with it. Then your abdomen is refilled with fresh dialysis solution, and the cycle is repeated. The process of draining and refilling is called an exchange.

Before your first treatment, a surgeon places a catheter into your abdomen or chest. The catheter tends to work better if there is adequate time-usually from 10 days to 2 or 3 weeks-for the insertion site to heal. Planning your dialysis access can improve treatment success. This catheter stays there permanently to help transport the dialysis solution to and from your abdomen.

Types of Peritoneal Dialysis

Three types of peritoneal dialysis are available.

- Continuous Ambulatory Peritoneal Dialysis (CAPD)
  CAPD requires no machine and can be done in any clean, well-lit place. With CAPD, your blood is always being cleaned. The dialysis solution passes from a plastic bag through the catheter and into your abdomen, where it stays for several hours with the catheter sealed. The time period that dialysis solution is in your abdomen is called the dwell time. Next, you drain the dialysis solution into an empty bag for disposal. You then refill your abdomen with fresh dialysis solution so the cleaning process can begin again. With CAPD, the dialysis solution stays in your abdomen for a dwell time of 4 to 6 hours, or more. The process of draining the used dialysis solution and replacing it with fresh solution takes about 30 to 40 minutes. Most people change the dialysis solution at least four times a day and sleep with solution in their abdomens at night. With CAPD, it's not necessary to wake up and perform dialysis tasks during the night.
- Continuous Cycler-assisted Peritoneal Dialysis (CCPD)
  CCPD uses a machine called a cycler to fill and empty your abdomen three to five times during the night while you sleep. In the morning, you begin one exchange with a dwell time that lasts the entire day. You may do an additional exchange in the middle of the afternoon without the cycler to increase the amount of waste removed and to reduce the amount of fluid left behind in your body.
- Combination of CAPD and CCPD
  If you weigh more than 175 pounds or if your peritoneum filters wastes slowly, you may need a combination of CAPD and CCPD to get the right dialysis dose. For example, some people use a cycler at night but also perform one exchange during the day. Others do four exchanges during the day and use a minicycler to perform one or more exchanges during the night. You'll work with your health care team to determine the best schedule for you.

Both types of peritoneal dialysis are usually performed by the patient without help from a partner. CAPD is a form of self-treatment that needs no machine. However, with CCPD, you need a machine to drain and refill your abdomen.

Possible Complications

The most common problem with peritoneal dialysis is peritonitis, a serious abdominal infection. This infection can occur if the opening where the catheter enters your body becomes infected or if contamination occurs as the catheter is connected or disconnected from the bags. Infection is less common in presternal catheters, which are placed in the chest. Peritonitis requires antibiotic treatment by your doctor.

To avoid peritonitis, you must be careful to follow procedures exactly and learn to recognize the early signs of peritonitis, which include fever, unusual color or cloudiness of the used fluid, and redness or pain around the catheter. Report these signs to your doctor or nurse immediately so that peritonitis can be treated quickly to avoid additional problems.

Diet for Peritoneal Dialysis

A peritoneal dialysis diet is slightly different from an in-center hemodialysis diet.
- You'll still need to limit salt and liquids, but you may be able to have more of each, compared with in-center hemodialysis.
- You must eat more protein.
- You may have different restrictions on potassium. You may even need to eat high-potassium foods.
- You may need to cut back on the number of calories you eat because there are calories in the dialysis fluid that may cause you to gain weight.

Your doctor and a dietitian who specializes in helping people with kidney failure will be able to help you plan your meals.

Pros and Cons

Each type of peritoneal dialysis (CAPD) or (CCPD) has advantages and disadvantages.

CAPD

Pros
- You can do it alone.
- You can do it at times you choose as long as you perform the required number of exchanges each day.
- You can do it in many locations.

- You don't need a machine.
- You won't have the ups and downs that many patients on hemodialysis feel.
- You don't need to travel to a center three times a week.

Cons

- It can disrupt your daily schedule.
- It is a continuous treatment, and all exchanges must be performed 7 days a week.

CCPD

Pros

- You can do it at night, mainly while you sleep.
- You are free from performing exchanges during the day.

Cons

- You need a machine.
- Your movement at night is limited by your connection to the cycler.

Working With Your Health Care Team

Questions you may want to ask:

- Is peritoneal dialysis the best treatment choice for me? Why? If yes, which type is best?
- How long will it take me to learn how to do peritoneal dialysis?
- What does peritoneal dialysis feel like?
- How will peritoneal dialysis affect my blood pressure?
- How will I know if I have peritonitis? How is it treated?
- As a peritoneal dialysis patient, will I be able to continue working?
- How much should I exercise?
- Where do I store supplies?
- How often do I see my doctor?
- Who will be on my health care team? How can these people help me?
- Whom do I contact with problems?
- With whom can I talk about finances, sexuality, or family concerns?
- How/where can I talk with other people who have faced this decision?

Dialysis Is Not a Cure

Hemodialysis and peritoneal dialysis are treatments that help replace the work your kidneys did. These treatments help you feel better and live longer, but they don't cure kidney failure. Although patients with kidney failure are now living longer than ever, over the years kidney disease can cause problems such as heart disease, bone disease, arthritis, nerve damage, infertility, and malnutrition. These problems won't go away with dialysis, but doctors now have new and better ways to prevent or treat them. You should discuss these complications and their treatments with your doctor.

Kidney Transplantation

Kidney transplantation surgically places a healthy kidney from another person into your body. The donated kidney does enough of the work that your two failed kidneys used to do to keep you healthy and symptom free.

A surgeon places the new kidney inside your lower abdomen and connects the artery and vein of the new kidney to your artery and vein. Your blood flows through the donated kidney, which makes urine, just like your own kidneys did when they were healthy. The new kidney may start working right away or may take up to a few weeks to make urine. Unless your own kidneys are causing infection or high blood pressure, they are left in place.

The transplantation process has many steps. First, talk with your doctor because transplantation isn't for everyone. You could have a condition that would make transplantation dangerous or unlikely to succeed.

You may receive a kidney from a deceased donor—a person who has recently died—or from a living donor. A living donor may be related or unrelated-usually a spouse or a friend. If you don't have a living donor, you're placed on a waiting list for a deceased donor kidney. The wait for a deceased donor kidney can be several years.

The transplant team considers three factors in matching kidneys with potential recipients. These factors help predict whether your body's immune system will accept the new kidney or reject it.

- Blood type. Your blood type (A, B, AB, or O) must be compatible with the donor's. Blood type is the most important matching factor.
- Human leukocyte antigens (HLAs). Your cells carry six important HLAs, three inherited from each parent. Family members are most likely to have a complete match. You may still receive a kidney if the HLAs aren't a complete match as long as your blood type is compatible with the organ donor's and other tests show no problems with matching.

- Cross-matching antigens. The last test before implanting an organ is the cross-match. A small sample of your blood will be mixed with a sample of the organ donor's blood in a tube to see if there's a reaction. If no reaction occurs, the result is called a negative cross-match, and the transplant operation can proceed.

How long you'll have to wait for a kidney varies. Because there aren't enough deceased donors for every person who needs a transplant, you must be placed on a waiting list. However, if a voluntary donor gives you a kidney, the transplant can be scheduled as soon as you're both ready. Avoiding the long wait is a major advantage of living donation.

The surgery takes 3 to 4 hours. The usual hospital stay is about a week. After you leave the hospital, you'll have regular follow-up visits.

In a living donation, the donor will probably stay in the hospital about the same amount of time. However, a new technique for removing a kidney for donation uses a smaller incision and may make it possible for the donor to leave the hospital in 2 to 3 days.

Between 85 and 90 percent of transplants from deceased donors are working 1 year after surgery. Transplants from living relatives often work better than transplants from unrelated or deceased donors because they're usually a closer match.

Possible Complications

Transplantation is the closest thing to a cure. But no matter how good the match, your body may reject your new kidney. A common cause of rejection is not taking medication as prescribed.

Your doctor will give you medicines called immunosuppressants to help prevent your body's immune system from attacking the kidney, a process called rejection. You'll need to take immunosuppressants every day for as long as the transplanted kidney is functioning. Sometimes, however, even these medicines can't stop your body from rejecting the new kidney. If this happens, you'll go back to some form of dialysis and possibly wait for another transplant.

Immunosuppressants weaken your immune system, which can lead to infections. Some medicines may also change your appearance. Your face may get fuller; you may gain weight or develop acne or facial hair. Not all patients have these problems, though, and diet and makeup can help.

Immunosuppressants work by diminishing the ability of immune cells to function. In some patients, over long periods of time, this diminished immunity can increase the risk of developing cancer. Some immunosuppressants can cause cataracts, diabetes, extra stomach acid, high blood pressure, and bone disease. When used over time, these drugs may also cause liver or kidney damage in a few patients.

Diet for Kidney Transplantation

Diet for transplant patients is less limited than it is for dialysis patients, although you may still have to cut back on some foods. Your diet will probably change as your medicines, blood values, weight, and blood pressure change.
- You may need to count calories. Your medicine may give you a bigger appetite and cause you to gain weight.
- You may have to eat less salt. Your medications may cause your body to retain sodium, leading to high blood pressure.

Pros and Cons

Kidney transplantation has advantages and disadvantages.

Pros
- A transplanted kidney works like a normal kidney.
- You may feel healthier and "more normal."
- You have fewer diet restrictions.
- You won't need dialysis.
- Patients who successfully go through the selection process have a higher chance of living a longer life.

Cons
- It requires major surgery.
- You may need to wait for a donor.
- Your body may reject the new kidney, so one transplant may not last a lifetime.
- You'll need to take immunosuppressants, which may cause complications.

Working With Your Health Care Team

Questions you may want to ask:
- Is transplantation the best treatment choice for me? Why?

- What are my chances of having a successful transplant?
- How do I find out whether a family member or friend can donate?
- What are the risks to a family member or friend who donates?
- If a family member or friend doesn't donate, how do I get placed on a waiting list for a kidney? How long will I have to wait?
- What symptoms does rejection cause?
- How long does a transplant work?
- What side effects do immunosuppressants cause?
- Who will be on my health care team? How can these people help me?
- With whom can I talk about finances, sexuality, or family concerns?
- How or where can I talk with other people who have faced this decision?

Refusing or Withdrawing from Treatment

For many people, dialysis and transplantation not only extend life but also improve quality of life. For others who have serious ailments in addition to kidney failure, dialysis may seem a burden that only prolongs suffering. You have the right to refuse or withdraw from dialysis. You may want to speak with your spouse, family, religious counselor, or social worker as you make this decision.

If you withdraw from dialysis treatments or refuse to begin them, you may live for a few days or for several weeks, depending on your health and your remaining kidney function. Your doctor can give you medicines to make you more comfortable during this time. You may start or resume your treatments if you change your mind about refusing dialysis.

Even if you're satisfied with your quality of life on dialysis, you should think about circumstances that might make you want to stop dialysis treatments. At some point in a medical crisis, you might lose the ability to express your wishes to your doctor. An advance directive is a statement or document in which you give instructions either to withhold treatment or to provide it, depending on your wishes and the specific circumstances.

An advance directive may be a living will, a document that details the conditions under which you would want to refuse treatment. You may state that you want your health care team to use all available means to sustain your life. Or you may direct that you be withdrawn from dialysis if you become permanently unresponsive or fall into a coma from which you won't awake. In addition to dialysis, other life-sustaining treatments you may choose or refuse include

- cardiopulmonary resuscitation (CPR)
- tube feedings
- mechanical or artificial respiration
- antibiotics
- surgery
- blood transfusions

Another form of advance directive is called a durable power of attorney for health care decisions or a health care proxy. In this type of advance directive, you assign a person to make health care decisions for you if you become unable to make them for yourself. Make sure the person you name understands your values and is willing to follow through on your instructions.

Each state has its own laws governing advance directives. You can obtain a form for an advance medical directive that's valid in your state from the National Hospice and Palliative Care Organization (see For More Information).

Paying for Treatment of Kidney Failure

Treatment for kidney failure is expensive, but Medicare and Medicaid pay much of the cost, usually up to 80 percent. Often, private insurance or state programs pay the rest.

Points to Remember

- Your kidneys filter wastes from your blood and regulate other functions of your body.
- When your kidneys fail, you need treatment to replace the work your kidneys normally perform.
- Your three choices for treatment are hemodialysis, peritoneal dialysis, and kidney transplantation.
- The choice you make will affect your diet, your ability to work, and other life style issues.
- You have the right to refuse or withdraw from treatment if you choose.
- Medicare and Medicaid pay much of the cost of treatment for kidney failure.

KIDNEY DISEASE AND CHILDREN

Kidney disease can affect children in various ways, ranging from treatable disorders without long-term consequences to life-threatening conditions. Acute kidney disease develops suddenly, lasts a short time, and can be serious with long-lasting consequences or may go away completely once the underlying cause has been treated. Chronic kidney disease (CKD) does not go away with treatment and tends to get worse over time. CKD eventually leads to kidney failure, described as end-stage kidney disease or ESRD when treated with a kidney transplant or blood-filtering treatments called dialysis.

Children with CKD or kidney failure face many challenges, which can include

- a negative self-image
- relationship problems
- behavior problems
- learning problems
- trouble concentrating
- delayed language skills development
- delayed motor skills development

Children with CKD may grow at a slower rate than their peers, and urinary incontinence—the loss of bladder control, which results in the accidental loss of urine—is common.

Read more in Facing the Challenges of Chronic Kidney Disease in Children at www.kidney.niddk.nih.gov.

Causes

Kidney disease in children can be caused by
- birth defects
- hereditary diseases
- infection
- nephrotic syndrome
- systemic diseases
- trauma
- urine blockage or reflux

From birth to age 4, birth defects and hereditary diseases are the leading causes of kidney failure. Between ages 5 and 14, kidney failure is most commonly caused by hereditary diseases, nephrotic syndrome, and systemic diseases. Between ages 15 and 19, diseases that affect the glomeruli are the leading cause of kidney failure, and hereditary diseases become less common.

Birth Defects

A birth defect is a problem that happens while a baby is developing in the mother's womb. Birth defects that affect the kidneys include renal agenesis (born withone kidney), renal dysplasia (one kidney doesn't function), and ectopic kidney (not in its usual place), to name a few. These defects are abnormalities of size, structure, or position of the kidneys.

In general, children with these conditions lead full, healthy lives. However, some children with renal agenesis or renal dysplasia are at increased risk for developing kidney disease.

Hereditary Diseases

Hereditary kidney diseases are illnesses passed from parent to child through the genes. One example is polycystic kidney disease (PKD), characterized by many grapelike clusters of fluid-filled cysts—abnormal sacs—that make both kidneys larger over time. These cysts take over and destroy working kidney tissue. Another hereditary disease is Alport syndrome, which is caused by a mutation in a gene for a type of protein called collagen that makes up the glomeruli. The condition leads to scarring of the kidneys. Alport syndrome generally develops in early childhood and is more serious in boys than in girls. The condition can lead to hearing and vision problems in addition to kidney disease.

Infection

Hemolytic uremic syndrome and acute post-streptococcal glomerulonephritis are kidney diseases that can develop in a child after an infection.

- Hemolytic uremic syndrome is a rare disease that is often caused by the Escherichia coli (E. coli) bacterium found in contaminated foods, such as meat, dairy products, and juice. Hemolytic uremic syndrome develops when E. coli bacteria lodged in the digestive tract make toxins that enter the bloodstream. The toxins start to destroy red blood cells and damage the lining of the blood vessels, including the glomeruli. Most children who get an E. coli infection have vomiting, stomach cramps, and bloody diarrhea for 2 to 3 days. Children who develop hemolytic uremic syndrome become pale, tired, and irritable. Hemolytic uremic syndrome can lead to kidney failure in some children.

- Post-streptococcal glomerulonephritis can occur after an episode of strep throat or a skin infection. The Streptococcus bacterium does not attack the kidneys directly; instead, the infection may stimulate the immune system to overproduce antibodies. Antibodies are proteins made by the immune system. The immune system protects people from infection by identifying and destroying bacteria, viruses, and other potentially harmful foreign substances. When the extra antibodies circulate in the blood and finally deposit in the glomeruli, the kidneys can be damaged. Most cases of post-streptococcal glomerulonephritis develop 1 to 3 weeks after an untreated infection, though it may be as long as 6 weeks. Post-streptococcal glomerulonephritis lasts only a brief time and the kidneys usually recover. In a few cases, kidney damage may be permanent.

Nephrotic Syndrome

Nephrotic syndrome is a collection of symptoms that indicate kidney damage. Nephrotic syndrome includes all of the following conditions:

- albuminuria—when a person's urine contains an elevated level of albumin, a protein typically found in the blood
- hyperlipidemia—higher-than-normal fat and cholesterol levels in the blood
- edema—swelling, usually in the legs, feet, or ankles and less often in the hands or face
- hypoalbuminemia—low levels of albumin in the blood

Nephrotic syndrome in children can be caused by the following conditions:

- Minimal change disease is a condition characterized by damage to the glomeruli that can be seen only with an electron microscope, which shows tiny details better than any other type of microscope. The cause of minimal change disease is unknown; some health care providers think it may occur after allergic reactions, vaccinations, and viral infections.
- Focal segmental glomerulosclerosis is scarring in scattered regions of the kidney, typically limited to a small number of glomeruli.

- Membranoproliferative glomerulonephritis is a group of autoimmune diseases that cause antibodies to build up on a membrane in the kidney. Autoimmune diseases cause the body's immune system to attack the body's own cells and organs.

Systemic Diseases

Systemic diseases, such as systemic lupus erythematosus (SLE or lupus) and diabetes, involve many organs or the whole body, including the kidneys:
- Lupus nephritis is kidney inflammation caused by SLE, which is an autoimmune disease.
- Diabetes leads to elevated levels of blood glucose, also called blood sugar, which scar the kidneys and increase the speed at which blood flows into the kidneys. Faster blood flow strains the glomeruli, decreasing their ability to filter blood, and raises blood pressure. Kidney disease caused by diabetes is called diabetic kidney disease. While diabetes is the number one cause of kidney failure in adults, it is an uncommon cause during childhood.

Trauma

Traumas such as burns, dehydration, bleeding, injury, or surgery can cause very low blood pressure, which decreases blood flow to the kidneys. Low blood flow can result in acute kidney failure.

Urine Blockage or Reflux

When a blockage develops between the kidneys and the urethra, urine can back up into the kidneys and cause damage. Reflux—urine flowing from the bladder up to the kidney—happens when the valve between the bladder and the ureter does not close all the way.

Diagnosis

A health care provider diagnoses kidney disease in children by completing a physical exam, asking for a medical history, and reviewing signs and symptoms. To confirm diagnosis, the health care provider may order one or more of the following tests:

Urine Tests

Dipstick test for albumin. The presence of albumin in urine is a sign that the kidneys may be damaged. Albumin in urine can be detected with a dipstick test performed on a urine sample. The urine sample is collected in a special container in a health care provider's office or a commercial facility and can be tested in the same location or sent to a lab for analysis. With a dipstick test, a nurse or technician places a strip of chemically treated paper, called a dipstick, into the person's urine sample. Patches on the dipstick change color when albumin is present in urine.

Urine albumin-to-creatinine ratio. A more precise measurement, such as a urine albumin-to-creatinine ratio, may be necessary to confirm kidney disease. Unlike a dipstick test for albumin, a urine albumin-to-creatinine ratio—the ratio between the amount of albumin and the amount of creatinine in urine—is not affected by variation in urine concentration.

Blood Test

Blood drawn in a health care provider's office and sent to a lab for analysis can be tested to estimate how much blood the kidneys filter each minute, called the estimated glomerular filtration rate or eGFR.

Imaging Studies

Imaging studies provide pictures of the kidneys. The pictures help the health care provider see the size and shape of the kidneys and identify any abnormalities.

Kidney Biopsy

Kidney biopsy is a procedure that involves taking a small piece of kidney tissue for examination with a microscope. Biopsy results show the cause of the kidney disease and extent of damage to the kidneys.

Treatment

Treatment for kidney disease in children depends on the cause of the illness. A child may be referred to a pediatric nephrologist—a doctor who specializes in treating kidney diseases and kidney failure in children—for treatment.

Children with a kidney disease that is causing high blood pressure may need to take medications to lower their blood pressure. Improving blood pressure can significantly slow the progression of kidney disease. The health care provider may prescribe

- angiotensin-converting enzyme (ACE) inhibitors, which help relax blood vessels and make it easier for the heart to pump blood
- angiotensin receptor blockers (ARBs), which help relax blood vessels and make it easier for the heart to pump blood
- diuretics, medications that increase urine output

Many children require two or more medications to control their blood pressure; other types of blood pressure medications may also be needed.

As kidney function declines, children may need treatment for anemia and growth failure. Anemia is treated with a hormone called erythropoietin, which stimulates the bone marrow to produce red blood cells. Children with growth failure may need to make dietary changes and take food supplements or growth hormone injections.

Children with kidney disease that leads to kidney failure must receive treatment to replace the work the kidneys do. The two types of treatment are dialysis and transplantation.

Birth Defects

Children with renal agenesis or renal dysplasia should be monitored for signs of kidney damage. Treatment is not needed unless damage to the kidney occurs. Ectopic kidney does not need to be treated unless it causes a blockage in the urinary tract or damage to the kidney. When a blockage is present, surgery may be needed to correct the position of the kidney for better drainage of urine. If extensive kidney damage has occurred, surgery may be needed to remove the kidney. Read more in Ectopic Kidney at www.kidney.niddk.nih.gov.

Hereditary Diseases

Children with PKD tend to have frequent urinary tract infections, which are treated with bacteria-fighting medications called antibiotics. PKD cannot be cured, so children with the condition receive treatment to slow the progression of kidney disease and treat the complications of PKD. Read more in Polycystic Kidney Disease at www.kidney.niddk.nih.gov.

Alport syndrome also has no cure. Children with the condition receive treatment to slow disease progression and treat complications until the kidneys fail. Read more in Glomerular Diseases Overview at www.kidney.niddk.nih.gov.

Infection

Treatment for hemolytic uremic syndrome includes maintaining normal salt and fluid levels in the body to ease symptoms and prevent further problems. A child may need a transfusion of red blood cells delivered through an intravenous (IV) tube. Some children may need dialysis for a short time to take over the work the kidneys usually do. Most children recover completely with no long-term consequences. Read more in Hemolytic Uremic Syndrome in Children at www.kidney.niddk.nih.gov.

Children with post-streptococcal glomerulonephritis may be treated with antibiotics to destroy any bacteria that remain in the body and with medications to control swelling and high blood pressure. They may also need dialysis for a short period of time. Read more about post-streptococcal glomerulonephritis in Glomerular Diseases Overview at www.kidney.niddk.nih.gov.

Nephrotic Syndrome

Nephrotic syndrome due to minimal change disease can often be successfully treated with corticosteroids. Corticosteroids decrease swelling and reduce the activity of the immune system. The dosage of the medication is decreased over time. Relapses are common; however, they usually respond to treatment. Corticosteroids are less effective in treating nephrotic syndrome due to focal segmental glomerulosclerosis or membranoproliferative glomerulonephritis. Children with these conditions may be given other immunosuppressive medications in addition to corticosteroids. Immunosuppressive medications prevent the body from making antibodies. Read more in Childhood Nephrotic Syndrome at www.kidney.niddk.nih.gov.

Systemic Diseases

Lupus nephritis is treated with corticosteroids and other immunosuppressive medications. A child with lupus nephritis may also be treated with blood pressure-lowering medications. In many cases, treatment is effective in completely or partially controlling lupus nephritis. Read more in Lupus Nephritis at www.kidney.niddk.nih.gov.

Diabetic kidney disease usually takes many years to develop. Children with diabetes can prevent or slow the progression of diabetic kidney disease by taking medications to control high blood pressure and maintaining normal blood glucose levels. Read more in Diabetic Kidney Disease at www.kidney.niddk.nih.gov.

Trauma

The types of trauma described above can be medically treated, though dialysis may be needed for a short time until blood flow and blood pressure return to normal.

Urine Blockage and Reflux

Treatment for urine blockage depends on the cause and severity of the blockage. In some cases, the blockage goes away without treatment. For children who continue to have urine blockage, surgery may be needed to remove the obstruction and restore urine flow. After surgery, a small tube, called a stent, may be placed in the ureter or urethra to keep it open temporarily while healing occurs. Read more in Urine Blockage in Newborns at www.kidney.niddk.nih.gov.

Treatment for reflux may include prompt treatment of urinary tract infections and long-term use of antibiotics to prevent infections until reflux goes away on its own. Surgery has also been used in certain cases. Read more in Vesicoureteral Reflux at www.kidney.niddk.nih.gov.

Diet and Nutrition

For children with CKD, learning about nutrition is vital because their diet can affect how well their kidneys work. Parents or guardians should always consult with their child's health care team before making any dietary changes. Staying healthy with CKD requires paying close attention to the following elements of a diet:

- Protein. Children with CKD should eat enough protein for growth while limiting high protein intake. Too much protein can put an extra burden on the kidneys and cause kidney function to decline faster. Protein needs increase when a child is on dialysis because the dialysis process removes protein from the child's blood. The health care team recommends the amount of protein needed for the child.
- Sodium. The amount of sodium children need depends on the stage of their kidney disease, their age, and sometimes other factors. The health care team may recommend limiting or adding sodium and salt to the diet.
- Potassium. Potassium levels need to stay in the normal range for children with CKD, because too little or too much potassium can cause heart and muscle problems. Children may need to stay away from some fruits and vegetables or reduce the number of servings and portion sizes to make sure they do not take in too much potassium. The health care team recommends the amount of potassium a child needs.
- Phosphorus. Children with CKD need to control the level of phosphorus in their blood because too much phosphorus pulls calcium from the bones, making them weaker and more likely to break. Too much phosphorus also can cause itchy skin and red eyes. As CKD progresses, a child may need to take a phosphate binder with meals to lower the concentration of phosphorus in the blood. Phosphorus is found in high-protein foods.
- Fluids. Early in CKD, a child's damaged kidneys may produce either too much or too little urine, which can lead to swelling or dehydration. As CKD progresses, children may need to limit fluid intake. The health care provider will tell the child and parents or guardians the goal for fluid intake.

Points to Remember

- Kidney disease can affect children in various ways, ranging from treatable disorders without long-term consequences to life-threatening conditions. Acute kidney disease develops suddenly, lasts a short time, and can be serious with long-lasting consequences, or may go away completely once the underlying cause has been treated.

- Chronic kidney disease (CKD) does not go away with treatment and tends to get worse over time.
- A health care provider diagnoses kidney disease in children by completing a physical exam, asking for a medical history, and reviewing signs and symptoms. To confirm diagnosis, the health care provider may order one or more tests.
- Treatment for kidney disease in children depends on the cause of the illness.
- Children with a kidney disease that is causing high blood pressure may need to take medications to lower their blood pressure. Improving blood pressure can significantly slow the progression of kidney disease. As kidney function declines, children may need treatment for anemia and growth failure.
- Children with kidney disease that leads to kidney failure must receive treatment to replace the work the kidneys do. The two types of treatment are dialysis and transplantation.
- For children with CKD, learning about nutrition is vital because their diet can affect how well their kidneys work. Parents or guardians should always consult with their child's health care team before making any dietary changes.

Hope through Research

The National Institute of Diabetes and Digestive and Kidney Diseases (NIDDK) conducts and supports research to help people with urologic diseases, including children. The NIDDK, in collaboration with the Eunice Kennedy Shriver National Institute of Child Health and Human Development and the National Heart, Lung, and Blood Institute, funded the formation of a cooperative agreement between two Clinical Coordinating Centers and a Data Coordinating Center to conduct a prospective epidemiological study of children with CKD. The primary goals of the Chronic Kidney Disease in Children Prospective Cohort Study (CKiD) are to

- determine the risk factors for decline in kidney function
- define how a progressive decline in kidney function affects neurocognitive function and behavior

- determine risk factors for cardiovascular disease
- assess growth failure and its associated morbidity

More information about the CKiD, funded under National Institutes of Health (NIH) clinical trial number NCT00327860, can be found at www.statepi.jhsph.edu/ckid.

6

Obesity

Obesity is described as having a body mass index (BMI) of 30 or higher, while a normal body weight rests between 18.5 and 24.9. Today, more than one third of U.S. adults—34.9% or 78.6 million—are obese.

Non-Hispanic blacks have the highest age-adjusted rates of obesity (47.8%) followed by Hispanics (42.5%), non-Hispanic whites (32.6%), and non-Hispanic Asians (10.8%). Obesity is higher among middle age adults, 40-59 years old (39.5%) than among younger adults, age 20-39 (30.3%) or adults over 60 or above (35.4%) adults.

Among men, obesity prevalence is generally similar at all income levels, however, among non-Hispanic black and Mexican-American men those with higher income are more likely to be obese than those with low income.

Higher income women are less likely to be obese than low income women, but most obese women are not low income.

There is no significant trend between obesity and education among men. Among women, however, there is a trend, those with college degrees are less likely to be obese compared with less educated women.

Obese individuals are at increased risk of diabetes, cardiovascular disease, hypertension and certain cancers, among other conditions.

Over the last 25 years, the prevalence of obesity increased in adults at all income and education levels.

The estimated annual medical cost of obesity in the U.S. is over $150 billion; the medical costs for people who are obese were $1,429 higher than those of normal weight.

DEFINING OVERWEIGHT AND OBESITY

Overweight and obesity are both labels for ranges of weight that are greater than what is generally considered healthy for a given height. The terms also identify ranges of weight that have been shown to increase the likelihood of certain diseases and other health problems.

For adults, overweight and obesity ranges are determined by using weight and height to calculate a number called the "body mass index" (BMI). BMI is used because, for most people, it correlates with their amount of body fat.

An adult who has a BMI between 25 and 29.9 is considered overweight.

An adult who has a BMI of 30 or higher is considered obese.

It is important to remember that although BMI correlates with the amount of body fat, BMI does not directly measure body fat. As a result, some people, such as athletes, may have a BMI that identifies them as overweight even though they do not have excess body fat.

Other methods of estimating body fat and body fat distribution include measurements of skinfold thickness and waist circumference, calculation of waist-to-hip circumference ratios, and techniques such as ultrasound, computed tomography, and magnetic resonance imaging (MRI).

HEALTH RISKS ASSOCIATED WITH OVERWEIGHT AND OBESITY

BMI is just one indicator of potential health risks associated with being overweight or obese. For assessing someone's likelihood of developing overweight- or obesity-related diseases, the National Heart, Lung, and Blood Institute guidelines recommend looking at two other predictors:

The individual's waist circumference (because abdominal fat is a predictor of risk for obesity-related diseases).

Other risk factors the individual has for diseases and conditions associated with obesity (for example, high blood pressure or physical inactivity).

CAUSES OF OBESITY

There are a variety of factors that play a role in obesity. This makes it a complex health issue to address. Behavior, environment, and genetic factors may have an effect in causing people to be overweight and obese.

Overweight and obesity result from an energy imbalance. This involves eating too many calories and not getting enough physical activity.

Body weight is the result of genes, metabolism, behavior, environment, culture, and socioeconomic status.

Behavior and environment play a large role causing people to be overweight and obese. These are the greatest areas for prevention and treatment actions.

Environment

People may make decisions based on their environment or community. For example, a person may choose not to walk to the store or to work because of a lack of sidewalks. Community, home, child care, school, health care, and workplace settings can all influence people's health decisions. Therefore, it is important to create environments in these locations that make it easier to engage in physical activity

Genetics

Science shows that genetics plays a role in obesity. Genes can directly cause obesity in disorders such as Bardet-Biedl syndrome and Prader-Willi syndrome. However genes do not always predict future health. Genes and behavior may both be needed for a person to be overweight. In some cases multiple genes may increase one's susceptibility for obesity and require outside factors; such as abundant food supply or little physical activity.

Diseases and Drugs

Some illnesses may lead to obesity or weight gain. These may include Cushing's disease, and polycystic ovary syndrome. Drugs such as steroids and some antidepressants may also cause weight gain. A doctor is the best source to tell you whether illnesses, medications, or psychological factors are contributing to weight gain or making weight loss hard.

HEALTH CONSEQUENCES

Research has shown that as weight increases to reach the levels referred to as "overweight" and "obesity," the risks for the following conditions also increases:

- Coronary heart disease
- Type 2 diabetes
- Cancers (endometrial, breast, and colon)
- Hypertension (high blood pressure)
- Dyslipidemia (for example, high total cholesterol or high levels of triglycerides)
- Stroke
- Liver and Gallbladder disease
- Sleep apnea and respiratory problems
- Osteoarthritis (a degeneration of cartilage and its underlying bone within a joint)
- Gynecological problems (abnormal menses, infertility)

ECONOMIC CONSEQUENCES

Overweight and obesity and their associated health problems have a significant economic impact on the U.S. health care system. Medical costs associated with overweight and obesity may involve direct and indirect costs. Direct medical costs may include preventive, diagnostic, and treatment services related to obesity. Indirect costs relate to morbidity and mortality costs. Morbidity costs are defined as the value of income lost from decreased productivity, restricted activity, absenteeism, and bed days. Mortality costs are the value of future income lost by premature death.

OBESITY IN CHILDREN

Childhood obesity prevalence remains high. Overall, obesity among our nation's young people, aged 2 to 19 years, has not changed significantly over the last ten years and remains at about 17 percent. However among 2-5 years old, obesity has declined based on CDC's National Health and Nutrition Examination Survey (NHANES) data.

Approximately 17% (or 12.7 million) of children and adolescents aged 2—19 years had obesity.

The prevalence of obesity among children aged 2 to 5 years decreased significantly from 13.9% in 2003-2004 to 8.4% in 2011-2012.

There are significant racial and age disparities in obesity prevalence among children and adolescents. In 2011-2012, obesity prevalence was higher among Hispanics (22.4%) and non-Hispanic black youth (20.2%) than non-Hispanic white youth (14.1%). The prevalence of obesity was lower in non-Hispanic Asian youth (8.6%) than in youth who were non-Hispanic white, non-Hispanic black or Hispanic.

In 2011-2012, 8.4% of 2- to 5-year-olds had obesity compared with 17.7% of 6- to 11-year-olds and 20.5% of 12- to 19-year-olds.

In children and adolescents aged 2 to 19 years, obesity was defined as a body mass index (BMI) at or above the 95th percentile of the sex-specific CDC BMI-for-age growth charts.

Childhood obesity is associated with adult head of household's education level for some children

Obesity prevalence differs among racial/ethnic groups and also varies by age, sex, and adult head of household's and education level.

Overall, obesity prevalence among children whose adult head of household completed college was approximately half that of those whose adult head of household did not complete high school (9% vs 19% among girls; 11% vs 21% among boys) in 1999–2010.

Among non-Hispanic white children, the lowest prevalence of obesity was observed among those whose adult head of household completed college; however, this was not the case for non-Hispanic black children.

Over time, the prevalence of obesity among girls whose adult head of household had not finished high school increased from 17% (1999–2002) to 23% (2007–2010), but decreased for girls whose adult head of household completed college from 11% (1999–2002) to 7% (2007–2010). There was not a similar finding among boys.

Childhood obesity among preschoolers is more prevalent among those from lower-income families

The prevalence of obesity among children aged 2–4 years from low-income households in 2011 varied by levels of income-to-poverty ratio,* which is a measure of household income.

Obesity prevalence was the highest among children in families with an income-to-poverty ratio of 100% or less (household income that is at or below the poverty threshold), followed by those in families with an income-to-poverty ratio of 101%–130%, and then found to be lower in children in families with an income-to-poverty ratio of 131% or larger (greater household income).

Obesity prevalence on the basis of family income among children from low-income households was:

- 14.2% among children in families with an income-to-poverty ratio of less than or equal to 50%.
- 14.5% among children in families with an income-to-poverty ratio of 51–100%.
- 13.4% among children in families with an income-to-poverty ratio of 101–130%.
- 12.4% among children in families with an income-to-poverty ratio of 131–150%.
- 11.8% among children in families with an income-to-poverty ratio of 151-185%.

There were differences in state-level childhood obesity estimates by income-to-poverty ratio. Income-to-poverty ratios reflect family income in relation to poverty threshold. The poverty level varies by family size, the number of related children, and the age of the head of household, but not by state. For example, a family of four with two children and an annual income of $22,811 were at the poverty level in 2011. For income-to-poverty ratios less than 100%, the family income is lower than the poverty threshold. When the ratio equals 100%, the income and poverty level are the same, and when the ratio is greater than 100%, the income is higher than the poverty level. A ratio of 130% indicates that family income was 30% above the poverty level.

Obesity prevalence is estimated by state and income-to-poverty ratio using information from the Pediatric Nutrition Surveillance System (PedNSS). PedNSS contains measured heights and weights, as well as other information from low-income children aged 2–4 years.

Obesity and extreme obesity rates decline among low-income preschool children

Obesity and extreme obesity among US low-income, preschool-aged children went down for the first time in recent years.

From 2003 through 2010, the prevalence of obesity decreased slightly from 15.21% to 14.94%. Similarly, the prevalence of extreme obesity decreased from 2.22% to 2.07%.

However, from 1998 through 2003, the prevalence of obesity increased from 13.05% to 15.21%, and the prevalence of extreme obesity increased from 1.75% to 2.22%.

Extreme obesity decreased among all racial groups except American Indians/Alaska Natives. The greatest decreases were among and Asian/Pacific Islander children and 2-year-old children. A child's weight status is determined using an age- and sex-specific percentile for BMI rather than the BMI categories used for adults because children's body composition varies by age and sex. The weight status of children is defined on the basis of the sex-specific smoothed percentile curves for BMI-for-age in the 2000 CDC growth Charts. Extreme obesity is defined as a BMI at or above the 120% of the 95th percentile for children of the same age and sex. For example, a 3-year-old boy of average height who weighs more than 44 pounds would be classified as extremely obese.

Significant Health Problems

Overweight and obesity in children are significant public health problems in the United States. The number of adolescents who are overweight has tripled since 1980 and the prevalence among younger children has more than doubled with 16 percent of children age 6-19 years overweight. Not only have the rates of overweight increased, but the heaviest children are markedly heavier than those in previous surveys.

Obesity disproportionately affects certain minority youth populations. NHANES found that African American and Mexican American adolescents ages 12-19 were more likely to be overweight, at 21 percent and 23 percent respectively, than non-Hispanic White adolescents (14 percent). In children 6-11 years old, 22 percent of Mexican American children were overweight, whereas 20 percent of African American children and 14 percent of non-Hispanic White children were overweight. In addition to the children and teens who were overweight in 1999-2002, another 15 percent were at risk of becoming overweight. In a national survey of American Indian children 5-18 years old, 39 percent were found to be overweight or at risk for overweight.

Being overweight during childhood and adolescence increases the risk of developing high cholesterol, hypertension, respiratory ailments, orthopedic problems, depression and type 2 diabetes as a youth. One disease of particular concern is Type 2 diabetes, which is linked to overweight and obesity and has increased dramatically in children and adolescents, particularly in American Indian, African American and Hispanic/Latino populations. The hospital costs alone associated with childhood obesity were estimated at $127 million during 1997–1999 (in 2001 constant U.S. dollars), up from $35 million during 1979–1981.

Looking at the long-term consequences, overweight adolescents have a 70 percent chance of becoming overweight or obese adults, which increases to 80 percent if one or more parent is overweight or obese. Obesity in adulthood increases the risk of diabetes, high blood pressure, high cholesterol, asthma, arthritis, and a general poor health status.

Factors of Childhood Obesity

The causes of childhood obesity are multi-factorial. Overweight in children and adolescents is generally caused by a lack of physical activity, unhealthy eating patterns resulting in excess energy intake, or a combination of the two. Genetics and social factors - socio-economic status, race/ethnicity, media and marketing, and the physical environment – also influence energy consumption and expenditure. Most factors of overweight and obesity do not work in isolation and solely targeting one factor may not going to make a significant impact on the growing problem.

To date, research has been unable to isolate the effects of a single factor due to the co-linearity of the variables as well as research constraints. Specific causes for the increase in prevalence of childhood obesity are not clear and establishing causality is difficult since longitudinal research in this area is limited. Such research must employ long study times to discern if there is an interaction of factors leading to an increase in the prevalence or the prevention of obesity during childhood and adolescence. Underreporting total food intake, misreporting of what was eaten, and over reporting physical activity are all likely potential biases that may affect the outcomes of studies in this area.

Nutrition and Eating Habits

It is difficult to correlate nutritional choices and childhood obesity using observational research. However, trend data suggest some changes in eating patterns and consumption that may be correlated with increases in obesity. In general, children and adolescents are eating more food away from home, drinking more sugar-sweetened drinks, and snacking more frequently. Convenience has become one of the main criteria for American's food choices today, leading more and more people to consume 'away-from-home' quick service or restaurant meals or to buy ready-to-eat, low cost, quickly accessible meals to prepare at home. The nutritional composition of children's diets as well as the number of calories consumed is of interest to determine the effect of food consumption on childhood obesity.

Below are notable trends gleaned from studies that used the USDA's Nationwide Food Consumption Survey and the Continuing Survey of Food Intakes by Individuals. These studies demonstrate changes in eating patterns among American youth that illustrate the complexity that exists relating food intake to the increased prevalence of obesity. Although the data is for the period from 1977 to 1996, it took eight years to analyze and the report published in 2005 is still the latest data available.

Children are getting more of their food away from home. Energy intake from away-from-home food sources increased from 20 to 32 percent from 1977-1978 to 1994-1996.

Daily total energy intake did not significantly increase for children 6-11, but did increase for adolescent girls and boys (ages 12-19 years) by 113 and 243 kilocalories, respectively.

Daily total energy intake that children derived from energy dense (high calorie) snacks increased by approximately 121 kilocalories between 1977 and 1996.

There has been a decline in breakfast consumption—especially for children of working mothers.

Portion sizes increased between 1977 and 1996. Average portion sizes increased for salty snacks from 1.0 oz to 1.6 oz and for soft drinks from 12.2 oz to 19.9 oz.

Other studies indicate that children are not eating the recommended servings of foods featured in the USDA food pyramid and that there have been significant changes in the types of beverages that children are consuming:

Only 21 percent of young people eat the recommended five or more servings of fruits and vegetables each day. Nearly half of all vegetable servings are fried potatoes.

Percent total energy from fat actually decreased between 1965 and 1996 for children, from 39 to 32 percent for total fat, and 15 to 12 percent for saturated fat. In 1994-1996, adolescent girls and boys only consumed 12 and 30 percent, respectively, of the Food Guide Pyramid's serving recommendations for dairy; and 18 and 14 percent, respectively, of the serving recommendations for fruit.

Soda consumption increased dramatically in the early to mid-1990s. Thirty-two percent of adolescent girls and 52 percent of adolescent boys consume three or more eight ounce servings of soda per day. Soft drink consumption for adolescent boys has nearly tripled, from seven to 22 oz. per day (1977-1978 to 1994). Children as young as seven months old are consuming soda.

Milk consumption has declined during the same period. In 1977-78, children age 6-11 drank four times as much milk as any other beverage. In 1994-1996 that decreased to 1.5 times as much milk as sugar sweetened beverages. In 1977-1978, adolescents drank 1.5 times as much milk as any other beverage and in 1996 they consumed twice as much sugar sweetened beverages as milk. Milk consumption decreased for adolescent boys and girls 37 and 30 percent respectively, between 1965 and 1996.

Several studies have been published that attempt to link children's diets with the onset of obesity. However, none have been able to show a causal link between diet and obesity. Two such studies include the Bogalusa Heart Study and a USDA Economic Research Service study.

The Bogalusa Heart Study analyzed children's eating patterns over two decades (1973-1994) using a series of seven cross-sectional surveys given to 1,584 ten year old children. The study discovered changes in children's eating patterns over this 20 year period including: increased incidence of missed breakfasts, increased numbers of children eating dinners outside the home, and increased snacking. No causal associations were found between changes in meal patterns and overweight status.

The USDA Economic Research Service study on fruit consumption indicated that higher fruit consumption is linked with a lower BMI in both adults and children. A large cohort of 3,064 children between the ages of 5 and 18 years were surveyed between 1994 and 1996 using the USDA's Continuing Survey of Food Intakes by Individuals (CSFII). The study hypothesized that people who incorporate nutrient-dense, low-fat foods into their diets like those found in fruits and vegetables will have a healthier BMI. However, the study only found a weak correlation between body weight and vegetable consumption.

Physical Inactivity and Sedentary Behaviors

Research indicates that a decrease in daily energy expenditure without a concomitant decrease in total energy consumption may be the underlying factor for the increase in childhood obesity. Physical activity trend data for children are limited, but cross sectional data indicates that one third of adolescents are not getting recommended levels of moderate or vigorous activity, 10 percent are completely inactive, and physical activity levels fall as adolescents age. This situation may actually be worse than these data describe. Activity measured by physical activity monitors tends to be significantly lower than what is reported on surveys.

Watching television, using the computer, and playing video games occupy a large percentage of children's leisure time, influencing their physical activity levels. It is estimated that children in the United States are spending 25 percent of their waking hours watching television and statistically, children who watch the most hours of television have the highest incidence of obesity. This trend is apparent not only because little energy is expended while viewing television but also because of the concurrent consumption of high-calorie snacks.

A recent examination of the Department of Education's Early Childhood Longitudinal Survey (ECLS-K) found that a one-hour increase in physical education per week resulted in a 0.31 point drop (approximately 1.8%) in body mass index among overweight and at-risk first grade girls. There was a smaller decrease for boys. The study concluded that expanding physical education in kindergarten to at least five hours per week could reduce the percentage of girls classified as overweight from 9.8 to 5.6 percent.

Currently, schools are decreasing the amount of free play or physical activity that children receive during school hours. Only about one-third of elementary children have daily physical education, and less than one-fifth have extracurricular physical activity programs at their schools. Daily enrollment in physical education classes among high school students decreased from 42 percent in 1991 to 25 percent in 1995, subsequently increasing slightly to 28 percent in 2003. Outside of school hours, only 39 percent of children ages 9-13 participate in an organized physical activity, although 77 percent engage in free-time physical activity.

Physical Environment

Experts have increasingly looked to the physical environment as a driver in the rapid increase of obesity in the United States. In urban and suburban areas, the developed environment can create obstacles to being physically active. In urban areas, space for outdoor recreation can be scarce, preventing kids from having a protected place to play; neighborhood crime, unattended dogs, or lack of street lighting may also inhibit children from being able to walk safely outdoors; and busy traffic can impede commuters from walking or biking to work as a means of daily exercise. Though few studies are available on the direct effects of the physical environment on physical activity, there are signs of the potential for improvement, evidenced by Toronto's 23 percent increase in bicycle use after the addition of bike lanes, and London's footpath use increase within the range of 34-101 percent (depending on location) as a result of improved lighting. There has been less research on the relationship between the physical environment and physical activity for children than for adults, however the findings for children appear to be consistent with those of the adult population. The percentage of trips to school that children walked declined from 20 percent in 1977 to 12 percent in 2001. Because children spend a substantial amount of time traveling to and from school, this may be an area in which to incorporate and increase physical activity into children's daily habits. Additionally, in-school environments have an impact on children's health. In a study of available school environments such as courts, fields and nets for physical activity in middle schools, environmental characteristics including the area type and size, supervision, temperature and organized activities explained 42 percent of the variance in the proportion of girls who were physically active and 59 percent of the variance in boys.

In suburban areas, the evolution of 'sprawl' can prevent residents from walking or biking and contributes to the great dependence on rising vehicle use. Suburban residents frequently lack adequate resources for physical recreation or sidewalks. In the first national study to establish a direct association between the form of the community and the health of the people who live there, analysts from Smart Growth America and the Centers for Disease Control and Prevention (CDC) found that "sprawl appears to have direct relationships to BMI and obesity." In the study, 488 counties were assigned a 'sprawl index' value, which ranged from 63 for the most sprawling county to 352 for the least sprawling county; the results showed that for a 50-point decrease in sprawl index value, the average BMI rose 0.17 points. Results also indicate that at the extremes, residents of the highest sprawling areas are likely to weigh six pounds more, on average, than residents of the most compact areas. Researchers reported that people in high sprawl counties were likely to weigh more, walk less, and have a higher prevalence of hypertension. Analysts agree that further research is required to determine direct causality between sprawl and health problems such as obesity, overweight, and hypertension.

Socio-Economic Status and Race/Ethnicity

Among adults, a negative relationship between socioeconomic status (SES) (e.g., parental income, parental education, occupation status) and being overweight or obese has been well established, however, the relationship appears weaker and less consistent in children. A number of studies find that SES is negatively associated with children being overweight or obese. It appears likely that the relationship between SES and obesity varies by race/ethnicity, such that the negative relationship is only apparent among White adolescents and is not apparent among Black or Mexican-American (and presumably other Latino) adolescents.

In other words, Black and Latino children from families with higher socioeconomic status are no less likely to be overweight or obese than those in families with lower socioeconomic status. Despite the more pronounced impact of SES among White children, they are substantially less likely to be overweight or obese than Black, Latino, or Native American children, who are disproportionately affected by obesity. In 1998, 21.5 percent of Black children and 21.8 percent of Latino children were overweight, while 12.3 percent of White children were. In a 2003 regional survey in the Aberdeen area, American Indian boys ages 5-17 years old had a prevalence of overweight at 22 percent and 18 percent for girls for the same age group. Furthermore, the prevalence at which obesity has been increasing in children in the recent years has been even more pronounced and rapid among minority children: between 1986 and 1998, obesity prevalence among African Americans and Hispanics increased 120 percent, as compared to a 50 percent increase among non-Hispanic Whites.

Findings from studies suggest that the effects of race/ethnicity and SES on the prevalence of childhood obesity cannot be individually determined because they are collinear. Therefore evidence is often inconsistent as a result of the difficulty of separating the overlapping factors. Furthermore, the relationship among race/ethnicity, SES, and childhood obesity may result from a number of underlying causes, including less healthy eating patterns (e.g., eating fewer fruits and vegetables, more saturated fats), engaging in less physical activity, more sedentary behavior, and cultural attitudes about body weight. Clearly these factors tend to co-occur and are likely to contribute jointly to differentials in increased risk of obesity in children.

Parental Influences

Numerous parental influences shape the eating habits of youth including; the choice of an infant feeding method, the foods they make available and accessible, the amount of time children are left unsupervised and their eating interactions with others in the social context. Several studies suggest that breastfeeding offers a small but consistent protective effect against obesity in children. This effect is most pronounced in early childhood. It has been hypothesized that exposure to complex sugars and fats contained in bottle formula influence "obesogenic factors" in infants, which predispose them to weight gain later on in life. A recent study postulated that breastfeeding may promote healthier eating habits because breastfed infants may eat until satiated, whereas bottle fed babies may be encouraged to eat until they have consumed all of the formula. Breast feeding also may expose babies to more variability in terms of nutrition and tastes since formula fed infants have experience with only a single flavor, whereas breastfed infants are exposed to a variety of flavors from the maternal diet that are transmitted through the milk. Research indicates that the perception of flavors in mother's milk is one of the human infant's earliest sensory experiences, and there is support for the idea that early experience with flavors has an effect on milk intake and the subsequent acceptance of a variety of foods.

Studies suggest that parental food preferences directly influence and shape those of their children. Parents who eat diets high in saturated fats also tend to have children that eat diets high in saturated fats. It is suspected that this observation is not merely due to the foods parents feed their children, but rather due to the preferences children develop through exposure to foods that their parents prefer early in their lives. Other studies have confirmed that availability and accessibility of fruits and vegetables was positively related to fruit and vegetable preferences and consumption by school children.

Additionally, child-feeding practices that control what and how much children eat can also affect their food preferences. Studies have determined that parents who attempt to encourage the consumption of food(s) may inadvertently cause children to dislike the food(s). Whereas parents that attempt to limit food(s) may actually promote increased preference and consumption of the limited food(s) in children.

Researchers also indicate that the social context in which a child is introduced to or has experiences with food is instrumental in shaping food preferences because the eating environment serves as a model for the developing child. For many children, eating is a social event that often times occurs in the presence of parents, other adults, older siblings and peers. In these contexts, children observe the behaviors and preferences of others around them. These role models have been found to have an influential effect on future food selection, especially when the model is similar to the child, or perceived as being powerful as in the case of older peers.

Over the last three decades there has been an increase in the number of dual income families as more women have entered the workforce and there has been an increase in the number of women serving as the sole supporter for their families. It has been hypothesized that increased rates and hours of parental employment may be correlated with the weight increases in American children (particularly for women because they still bear the bulk of the responsibility of caring for children). Studies have demonstrated that children in single-parent families are more likely to be overweight or obese than children in two-parent families and that the rise in women working outside the home coincides with the rise in childhood weight problems. Several potential mechanisms have been proposed to explain this phenomenon including the following:

Constraints on parent's time potentially contribute to children's weight problems, as working parents probably rely more heavily than non-working parents on prepared, processed, and fast foods, which generally have high calorie, high fat, and low nutritional content.

Children left unsupervised after school may make poor nutritional choices and engage in more sedentary activities.

Child care providers may not offer as many opportunities for physical activity and may offer less nutritious food alternatives.

Unsupervised children may spend a great deal of time indoors, perhaps due to safety concerns, watching TV or playing video games rather than engaging in more active outdoor pursuits.

In short, the recent social and economic changes in American society have encouraged the consumption of excess energy and have had a detrimental effect on energy expenditure among youth. These changes have impacted the foods available in the homes, the degree of influence parents have when children make food selections and has led to increases in sedentary behaviors among youth.

Genetics

There is an abundance of evidence that supports genetic susceptibility as an important risk factor for obesity. Evidence from twin, adoption and family studies strongly suggests that biological relatives exhibit similarities in maintenance of body weight, and that heredity contributes between five and 40 percent of the risk for obesity. Other studies indicate that 50-70 percent of a person's BMI and degree of adiposity (fatness) is determined by genetic influences and that there is a 75 percent chance that a child will be overweight if both parents are obese, and a 25-50 percent chance if just one parent is obese.

Though this relationship is well established, the role of genetics in obesity is complex. While over 250 obesity-associated genes have been identified, there is no one 'smoking gun'. Cases of monogenic obesity and related syndromes do exist, but they are extremely rare and only account for a small number of those who are overweight and obese. To date only six single gene specific defects that result in obesity have been found, and appear to affect fewer than 150 people.[94] Genetic susceptibility to obesity in most cases is due to multiple genes that interact with environmental and behavioral factors. Simply having a genetic predisposition to obesity does not guarantee that an individual will develop the disease.

It must also be noted that the recent increases in weight observed in the American population are not correlated with genetics. Despite the strong influence that genetics has on obesity, the genetic composition of a population does not change rapidly, and moreover, the characteristics of the American population have not dramatically changed. Therefore, increases in the incidence and prevalence rates of obesity in the US are likely due to behavioral or environmental factors, which have interacted with genes, and not the effects of genetics alone.

Advertising and Marketing

There has been considerable debate over whether exposure to food advertising affects incidence rates of childhood obesity. While the positive correlation between the hours of television viewed, body mass index, and obesity incidence has been documented, the exact mechanisms through which this occurs are still being investigated. It has been estimated that the average child currently views more than 40,000 commercials on television each year, a sharp increase from 20,000 in the 1970s. Moreover, an accumulated body of research reveals that more than 50 percent of television advertisements directed at children promote foods and beverages such as candy, convenience foods, snack foods, sugar sweetened beverages and sweetened breakfast cereals that are high in calories and fat and low in fiber and nutrient density. The statistics on food advertising to children indicate that:

Annual sales of foods and beverages to young consumers exceeded $27 billion in 2002.

Food and beverage advertisers collectively spend $10 to $12 billion annually to reach children and youth: more than $1 billion is spent on media advertising to children (primarily on television); more than $4.5 billion is spent on youth-targeted public relations; and $3 billion is spent on packaging designed for children.

Fast food outlets spend $3 billion in television ads targeted to children.

A growing body of research suggests that there may be a link between exposure to food advertising and the increasing rates of obesity among youth. In the 1970s and 1980s a number of experimental studies were conducted that demonstrated young children (under age eight) were much more likely than older children to believe that television advertisements were telling the truth; and that exposure to television advertisements influenced the food choices among children (enticing them to choose more sugary foods instead of natural options) which increased requests to parents for high sugar foods they saw advertised. Though many of these studies did find significant correlations between advertising and behavioral change, the reliability of these findings are equivocal because many of the studies use small sample sizes, and some of them are more than 25 years old.

A recent literature review by Kaiser Family Foundation highlighted a number of studies that suggested that advertising influenced dietary and other food choices in children, which likely contributed to energy imbalance and weight gain. One study found that among children as young as three, the amount of weekly television viewing was significantly related to their caloric intake as well as requests and parental purchases of specific foods they saw advertised on television. Several other studies found that the amount of time children spent watching TV was correlated with how often they requested products at the grocery store and their product and brand preferences.

Exposure to food advertising on television can affect eating behavior, stimulating energy intake from a range of advertised foods and exaggerating unhealthy choices in foods. The excess intake of calories above the daily expenditure of energy leads to weight gain and can eventually lead to obesity. The main components of this equation are energy intake (diet) and energy expenditure (physical activity, metabolic rate, etc.).

The nutrition and physical activity habits of U.S. children have been changing over the past 40 years. Research shows some correlation of these changes to the increases in obesity levels in children. The physical environment, socio-economic status and race/ethnicity, family structure, genetics, and advertising may also influence diet and levels of physical activity among American youth.

Available research shows that there are a number of root causes of obesity in children. Selecting one or two main causes or essential factors is next to impossible given the current data, because the potential influences of obesity are multiple and intertwined. There are large gaps in knowledge, limiting the ability to pinpoint a particular cause and determine the most effective ways to combat childhood obesity. Another research gap stems from lack of a prospective longitudinal study that links dietary and other behavior patterns to development of obesity. Another complication of current data is that there is a need for more precise and reliable measures of dietary intake and activity levels, as individual recall of events and diet are not the most dependable sources for information.

When thinking about early prevention of obesity, it is essential that more is understood about how genetics is involved and how the genes are triggered or react to environmental changes and stimuli. Additionally, research is only beginning to explain how taste preferences develop, their biochemical underpinnings and how this information may be useful in curbing childhood weight gain.

Primary prevention is not an option for many children who are already overweight. Research on successful interventions for children who are overweight or at risk of becoming overweight is extremely important to effectively reduce childhood obesity in this country. Overall, research has just begun to scratch the surface in elucidating the causes of obesity in children. Filling in the knowledge gaps will take time, as implementing some of the study designs that will best illuminate the complex interactions are time consuming and costly. However the fundamentals are clear, to stay healthy, eat a balanced diet and devote adequate time to physical activity.

HEALTHY EATING FOR A HEALTHY WEIGHT

A healthy lifestyle involves many choices. Among them, choosing a balanced diet or healthy eating plan. According to the Dietary Guidelines for Americans 2010, a healthy eating plan:

- Emphasizes fruits, vegetables, whole grains, and fat-free or low-fat milk and milk products
- Includes lean meats, poultry, fish, beans, eggs, and nuts
- Is low in saturated fats, trans fats, cholesterol, salt (sodium), and added sugars
- Stays within your daily calorie needs

A healthy eating plan that helps you manage your weight includes a variety of foods you may not have considered. If "healthy eating" makes you think about the foods you can't have, try refocusing on all the new foods you can eat.

Fresh fruits — don't think just apples or bananas. All fresh fruits are great choices. Be sure to try some "exotic" fruits, too. How about a mango? Or a juicy pineapple or kiwi fruit! When your favorite fresh fruits aren't in season, try a frozen, canned, or dried variety of a fresh fruit you enjoy. One caution about canned fruits is that they may contain added sugars or syrups. Be sure and choose canned varieties of fruit packed in water or in their own juice.

Fresh vegetables — try something new. You may find that you love grilled vegetables or steamed vegetables with an herb you haven't tried like rosemary. You can sauté (panfry) vegetables in a non-stick pan with a small amount of cooking spray. Or try frozen or canned vegetables for a quick side dish — just microwave and serve. When trying canned vegetables, look for vegetables without added salt, butter, or cream sauces. Commit to going to the produce department and trying a new vegetable each week.

Calcium-rich foods — you may automatically think of a glass of low-fat or fat-free milk when someone says "eat more dairy products." But what about low-fat and fat-free yogurts without added sugars? These come in a wide variety of flavors and can be a great dessert substitute for those with a sweet tooth.

A new twist on an old favorite — if your favorite recipe calls for frying fish or breaded chicken, try healthier variations using baking or grilling. Maybe even try a recipe that uses dry beans in place of higher-fat meats. Ask around or search the internet and magazines for recipes with fewer calories — you might be surprised to find you have a new favorite dish!

Healthy eating is all about balance. You can enjoy your favorite foods even if they are high in calories, fat or added sugars. The key is eating them only once in a while, and balancing them out with healthier foods and more physical activity. Some general tips for comfort foods:

Eat them less often. If you normally eat these foods every day, cut back to once a week or once a month. You'll be cutting your calories because you're not having the food as often.

Eat smaller amounts. If your favorite higher-calorie food is a chocolate bar, have a smaller size or only half a bar.

Try a lower-calorie version. Use lower-calorie ingredients or prepare food differently. For example, if your macaroni and cheese recipe uses whole milk, butter, and full-fat cheese, try remaking it with non-fat milk, less butter, light cream cheese, fresh spinach and tomatoes. Just remember to not increase your portion size.

The point is, you can figure out how to include almost any food in your healthy eating plan in a way that still helps you lose weight or maintain a healthy weight.

PHYSICAL ACTIVITY FOR A HEALTHY WEIGHT

Regular physical activity is important for good health, and it's especially important if you're trying to lose weight or to maintain a healthy weight.

When losing weight, more physical activity increases the number of calories your body uses for energy or "burns off." The burning of calories through physical activity, combined with reducing the number of calories you eat, creates a "calorie deficit" that results in weight loss.

Most weight loss occurs because of decreased caloric intake. However, evidence shows the only way to maintain weight loss is to be engaged in regular physical activity.

Most importantly, physical activity reduces risks of cardiovascular disease and diabetes beyond that produced by weight reduction alone.

Physical activity also helps to:

- Maintain weight.
- Reduce high blood pressure.
- Reduce risk for type 2 diabetes, heart attack, stroke, and several forms of cancer.
- Reduce arthritis pain and associated disability.

- Reduce risk for osteoporosis and falls.
- Reduce symptoms of depression and anxiety.

When it comes to weight management, people vary greatly in how much physical activity they need. Here are some guidelines to follow:

To maintain your weight: Work your way up to 150 minutes of moderate-intensity aerobic activity, 75 minutes of vigorous-intensity aerobic activity, or an equivalent mix of the two each week. Strong scientific evidence shows that physical activity can help you maintain your weight over time. However, the exact amount of physical activity needed to do this is not clear since it varies greatly from person to person. It's possible that you may need to do more than the equivalent of 150 minutes of moderate-intensity activity a week to maintain your weight.

To lose weight and keep it off: You will need a high amount of physical activity unless you also adjust your diet and reduce the amount of calories you're eating and drinking. Getting to and staying at a healthy weight requires both regular physical activity and a healthy eating plan.

What do moderate- and vigorous-intensity mean?

Moderate: While performing the physical activity, if your breathing and heart rate is noticeably faster but you can still carry on a conversation — it's probably moderately intense. Examples include:

- Walking briskly (a 15-minute mile).
- Light yard work (raking/bagging leaves or using a lawn mower).
- Light snow shoveling.
- Actively playing with children.
- Biking at a casual pace.

Vigorous: Your heart rate is increased substantially and you are breathing too hard and fast to have a conversation, it's probably vigorously intense. Examples include:

- Jogging/running.
- Swimming laps.
- Rollerblading/inline skating at a brisk pace.
- Cross-country skiing.
- Most competitive sports (football, basketball, or soccer).
- Jumping rope.

7

Respiratory Diseases

Asthma, bronchitis, emphysema, chronic obstructive pulmonary disease (COPD), and obstructive sleep apnea (OSA) are a significant public health burden to the United States. Specific methods of detection, intervention, and treatment exist that may reduce this burden. Certain other important respiratory diseases, such as respiratory distress syndromes, sarcoidosis, and chronic sinusitis, are difficult to define, detect, prevent, or treat.

Asthma and COPD are among the 10 leading chronic conditions causing restricted activity. After chronic sinusitis, asthma is the most common cause of chronic illness in children. Methods are available to treat these respiratory diseases and promote respiratory health.

In the United States, tobacco smoke is a key factor in the development and progression of COPD, although exposure to air pollutants in the home and workplace, genetic factors, and respiratory infections also play a role. In the developing world, indoor air quality is thought to play a larger role in the development and progression of COPD than it does in the United States.

Chronic lower respiratory disease, primarily COPD, was the third leading cause of death in the United States. Fifteen million Americans report that they have been diagnosed with COPD. More than 50% of adults with low pulmonary function were not aware that they had COPD, therefore the actual number may be higher. The following groups were more likely to report COPD:

- People aged 65–74 years.
- Non-Hispanic whites.
- Women.
- Individuals who were unemployed, retired, or unable to work.

- Individuals with less than a high school education.
- People with lower incomes.
- Individuals who were divorced, widowed, or separated.
- Current or former smokers.
- Those with a history of asthma.

PREVENTION AND TREATMENT

Avoid inhaling tobacco smoke, home and workplace air pollutants, and respiratory infections to prevent developing COPD. Early detection of COPD might change its course and progress. A simple test, called spirometry can be used to measure pulmonary—or lung—function and detect COPD in anyone with breathing problems.

Treatment of COPD requires a careful and thorough evaluation by a physician. COPD treatment can alleviate symptoms, decrease the frequency and severity of exacerbations, and increase exercise tolerance. For those who smoke, the most important aspect of treatment is smoking cessation. Avoiding tobacco smoke and removing other air pollutants from the patient's home or workplace are also important. Symptoms such as coughing or wheezing can be treated with medication. Pulmonary rehabilitation is an individualized treatment program that teaches COPD management strategies to increase quality of life. Plans may include breathing strategies, energy-conserving techniques, and nutritional counseling. The flu can cause serious problems in people with COPD. Vaccination during flu season is recommended and respiratory infections should be treated with antibiotics, if appropriate. Patients who have low blood oxygen levels are often given supplemental oxygen.

ASTHMA

Asthma is a serious and growing health problem. An estimated 14.9 million persons in the United States have asthma. The number of people with asthma increased by 102 percent between 1979-80 and 1993-94.

Asthma is responsible for about 500,000 hospitalizations, 5,000 deaths, and 134 million days of restricted activity a year. Yet most of the problems caused by asthma could be averted if persons with asthma and their health care providers managed the disease according to established guidelines. Effective management of asthma comprises four major components: controlling exposure to factors that trigger asthma episodes, adequately managing asthma with medicine, monitoring the disease by using objective measures of lung function, and educating asthma patients to become partners in their own care. Such prevention efforts are essential to interrupt the progression from disease to functional limitation and disability and to improve the quality of life for persons with asthma.

In 1996, asthma was the 10th most common principal diagnosis in emergency department (ED) visits. Among diseases commonly seen in outpatient departments, asthma was the ninth most frequent diagnosis in 1996. In 1995, some 9 million physician office visits were made for asthma. From 1990 to 1992, persons with asthma spent an estimated 64 million days in bed because of asthma, ranking asthma as the fourth highest chronic condition. The proportion of people with asthma who are limited in activity increased slightly from 19.4 percent in 1986-88 to 19.6 percent in 1994-96.

Direct medical expenditures for asthma amounted to $3.64 billion in 1990, and indirect economic losses accounted for an additional $2.6 billion. Of direct medical care costs, approximately 57 percent was spent on hospitalizations ($1.6 billion), outpatient hospital visits ($190 million), and emergency department visits ($295 million). Physician-related services accounted for 14 percent of the total expenditures, including $347 million for outpatient services. Prescription medications represented 30 percent of direct medical costs. Such facts highlight the significant cost of hospital care for asthma, compared to the more frequently used and less costly outpatient and pharmaceutical services.

Indirect costs—nonmedical economic losses such as days missed from work or school, caregiver costs, travel and waiting time, early retirement due to disability, and premature death—account for slightly less than 50 percent of the total costs of asthma. Data suggest that the uneven distribution of costs of asthma relates to nonscheduled acute or emergency care, indicating poor asthma management and suboptimal outcomes.

Environmental and occupational factors contribute to illness and disability from asthma. Decreases in lung function and a worsening of asthma have been associated with exposure to allergens, indoor pollutants (for example, tobacco smoke), and ambient air pollutants (for example, ozone, sulfur dioxide, nitrogen dioxide, acid aerosols, and particulate matter). Approximately 25 percent of children in the United States live in areas that exceed the Federal Government's standard for ozone. Occupational factors cause or trigger asthma episodes in 5 to 30 percent of adults with the disease. Environmental factors are associated with upper respiratory infections, which contribute to illness and disability in children and adults.

Disparities within the U.S. population, the health, economic, and social burdens of asthma vary. Disproportionate rates of death, hospitalization, emergency room use, and disability from asthma occur in specific age, gender, racial, and ethnic groups.

While the number of adults with asthma is greater than the number of children with asthma, the asthma rate is rising more rapidly in preschool-aged children than in any other group. In 1995, the rate of self-reported asthma among children and adolescents under age 18 years was 7.5 percent, compared to 5.7 percent among the general population. The rates were higher in boys under age 18 years than in girls in the same age group. The rates of self-reported asthma were higher for women (6.7 percent) than men (5.2 percent) and higher for African Americans (6.7 percent) than whites (5.6 percent). Among adults, women of all races have higher rates of illness and death from asthma than men.

Death from asthma is 2 to 6 times more likely to occur among African Americans and Hispanics than among whites.1 Although the number of deaths annually from asthma is low compared to other chronic diseases, the death rate for children aged 5 to 14 years and young adults aged 15 to 24 years doubled from 1979-80 to 199395 (from 1.5 to 3.7 deaths per million children aged 5 to 14 years and 2.8 to 6.3 deaths per million persons aged 15 to 34 years, respectively). In 1993-95, death rates are slightly higher overall in women than in men.

Rates of hospitalization for asthma demonstrate similar variations. Rates for African Americans are almost triple those for whites. Rates are higher among women than among men. Asthma hospitalization rates have increased dramatically among children under age 5 years. From 1980 to 1993, the rate increased from 36 to 65 children hospitalized per 10,000 children under age 1 year. Some of this increase may be related to changes in diagnostic practices and changes in coding and reimbursement, but a large portion represents a true increase in illness and disability.

In the inner city, patients frequently use EDs for asthma care. In 1993 and 1994, African Americans were 4 times more likely than whites to visit an ED because of asthma. Asthma patients in general and high-risk inner-city patients—in particular, those with a history of severe asthma who were hospitalized or visited the ED for asthma within the previous 2 years—need to be able to recognize the signs and symptoms of uncontrolled asthma and know how to respond appropriately.

The economic burden of asthma disproportionately affects patients with severe disease. Socioeconomic status, particularly poverty, appears to be an important contributing factor to asthma illness, disability, and death. In the United States, the rate of asthma cases for nonwhites is only slightly higher than for whites, yet the death, hospitalization, and ED visit rates for nonwhites are more than twice those for whites. Although reasons for these differences are unclear, they likely result from multiple factors: high levels of exposure to environmental tobacco smoke, pollutants, and environmental allergens (for example, house dust mites, cockroach particles, cat and dog dander, and possibly rodent dander and mold); a lack of access to quality medical care; and a lack of financial resources and social support to manage the disease effectively on a long-term basis. Research into the role of socioeconomic factors is needed to identify additional prevention opportunities.

Scientific research has led to greater asthma control than was available in the early 1980s. Effective management of asthma includes four components: avoiding or controlling the factors that may make asthma worse (for example, environmental and occupational allergens and irritants), taking appropriate medications tailored to the severity of the disease, objective monitoring of the disease by the patient and the health care professional, and actively involving the patient in managing the disease. Effective asthma management reduces the need for hospitalizations and urgent care visits (in either an ED or physician's office) and enables patients to enjoy normal activities.

Advances in human genetics related to asthma are expected to provide better information about the contribution of genetic variation to the development of disease when people are exposed to certain environmental factors. The use of this genetic information will improve targeted disease prevention and health management strategies for respiratory diseases.

Patient education is one of four components of effective asthma management. Patients who are taught asthma self-management skills are able to manage and control their disease better than patients who do not receive education.6 Patients need to learn to work with health care providers to optimize asthma care. Thus, both patients and health care providers need to be trained and educated on effective asthma management. Health outcomes for asthma—illness, disability, quality of life, and death—

are related directly to the actions of health care professionals and patients. The National Asthma Education and Prevention Program (NAEPP) provides guidelines for diagnosis and management which should be incorporated into the curricula of health professional schools. Currently, there are no national data systems for tracking the training of health care providers in asthma management. It represents an important research and data collection agenda for the coming decade. In addition, research to identify the primary causes of development of asthma is a high priority. Such research can provide a scientific basis for efforts to prevent the development of asthma.

To control asthma effectively, asthma patients, particularly those on daily medication, need an action plan developed under their physician's guidance. The plan spells out when and how to take medicines correctly, as well as what to do when asthma worsens. The treatment of persistent asthma emphasizes daily long-term therapy aimed at the underlying inflammation and preventing symptoms, rather than relying solely on treating symptoms with short-acting inhaled medication, such as a short-acting beta agonist medication. Use of more than one canister of the medication per month is an indication of uncontrolled asthma and the need to start or increase long-term preventive therapy. Patients also need to work with health care providers during follow-up visits, particularly after being hospitalized, to make sure they understand and are able to follow the long-term management plan.

Working with local community groups to mobilize community resources for a comprehensive, culturally and linguistically competent approach to controlling asthma among high-risk populations is a priority. From a community-based perspective, States need to track occupational and environmental factors that cause or trigger asthma episodes. Such surveillance efforts should include collecting State-based data on the proportion of the population with asthma and monitoring occupational and environmental exposures and their impact on illness and disability related to asthma. Efforts directed to improving the environmental management of asthma also include reducing exposure to allergens and irritants, such as environmental tobacco smoke, and outdoor air pollution from ozone, sulfur dioxide, and particulate diesel matter.

Professional organizations, lay volunteer groups, Federal agencies, and the private sector have worked together and with NAEPP to implement a spectrum of asthma programs at national and local community levels. For example, numerous publications, media campaigns, and conferences target different audiences. Intensified efforts are planned to reach primary care providers, patients, and school personnel. A high-level work group convened by the U.S. Department of Health and Human Services assessed the most urgent needs for tackling the growing problem of asthma. The work group's department-wide strategic plan, Action Against Asthma, identified opportunities and presented a coordinated approach for improving asthma prevention and management.

CHRONIC OBSTRUCTIVE PULMONARY DISEASE

COPD includes chronic bronchitis and emphysema—both of which are characterized by irreversible airflow obstruction and often exist together. Similar to asthma, COPD may be accompanied by an airway hyper responsiveness. Most patients with COPD have a history of cigarette smoking. COPD worsens over time with continued exposure to a causative agent—usually tobacco smoke or sometimes a substance in the workplace or environment.

COPD occurs most often in older people. As much as 10 percent of the population 65 years of age and over is estimated to have COPD. COPD has a major impact on health care, illness, disability, and death in the older population, and the magnitude of the problem is growing. Since 1980, the prevalence and age-adjusted death rate for COPD increased more than 30 percent. Most of the increase occurred in people over age 65 years. Taking into account the expected aging of the U.S. population over the next 10 to 30 years as well as the improved management of other smoking-related diseases, any decline in the proportion of persons with COPD is unlikely without substantial changes in risk factors, mainly reductions in cigarette smoking. This is important for both men and women, given the modest decline in cigarette smoking rates from 1990 to 1995.

Between 80 and 90 percent of COPD is attributable to cigarette smoking. However, not all smokers develop COPD, and not all patients with COPD are smokers or have smoked in the past. Individual susceptibility to the adverse health effects of cigarette smoke on the lung appears to vary within the general population. Some 10 to 15 percent of smokers show a rate of decline in lung function that will result in COPD with severe disability. Smoking cessation is the only treatment that slows the decline. Susceptible smokers who stop smoking do not regain lost lung function, but the rate of loss will return to what is normal for a nonsmoker.

How cigarette smoking causes COPD is an active area of research. The development of COPD—in particular, emphysema—is thought to be due to a chemical imbalance in the lungs caused by cigarette smoke. In some individuals, emphysema occurs because of a genetic deficiency. Emphysema due to genetic deficiency, called familial emphysema, occurs even in nonsmokers, but smoking hastens its occurrence. Familial emphysema probably accounts for less than 5 percent of all cases of COPD.

Smoking and occupational exposures together cause respiratory diseases and lung cancer. Miners, firefighters, metal workers, grain handlers, cotton workers, paper mill workers, agricultural workers, construction workers who handle cement, and others employed in occupations associated with prolonged exposure to dusts, fumes, or gases develop significant airflow obstruction, coughing, phlegm, dyspnea, wheezing, and reduced lung function.

Population studies have shown that chronic exposure to air pollution has an independent adverse effect on lung function. A multi-year study of the respiratory effects of long-term exposure to environmental tobacco smoke and air pollution reported that both long-term ozone and childhood exposure to maternal tobacco smoke were associated with diminished lung function in college students. Viral infections also may contribute to susceptibility to COPD, and they are considered to play a role in the onset of airflow obstruction.

The direct costs of health care services and indirect costs through loss of productivity related to COPD amounted to $26 billion in 1998. About 14 million persons in the United States have COPD—about 12.5 million have chronic bronchitis and 1.9 million have emphysema. Emphysema has not increased, but since 1980, cases of chronic bronchitis increased 75 percent.

Reliable statistics are not as available for COPD total cases, illness, disability, or death in African Americans, Hispanics, and other ethnic groups as for whites. From 1982 to 1984, the proportion of adults with COPD was 6.2 percent among whites and 3.2 percent among African Americans. In 1982, the age-adjusted COPD death rate for whites was 16.6 deaths per 1,000 population and 12.8 deaths per 1,000 for African Americans. Among the Hispanic groups studied, Puerto Ricans demonstrated a higher proportion of chronic bronchitis (2.9 percent) than Mexican Americans (1.7 percent) or Cuban Americans (1.7 percent).

In 1995, the proportion of the population with COPD was 5 percent in men aged 45 to 64 years and 11 percent in men aged 65 years or older. The proportion was 10 percent in women aged 45 to 64 years and 9 percent in women aged 65 to 74 years.

Death from COPD is more common in men than in women, and the death rate increases steeply with age. Men and women have similar COPD death rates before age 55 years, but the rate for men rises thereafter. At age 70 years, the rate for men is more than double that for women, and at age 85 years and older, the COPD death rate for men is 3.5 times that for women. The proportion was 8 percent for whites aged 45 to 64 years and 10 percent for whites aged 65 years and older. The proportion of African Americans with COPD was 6 percent for those aged 45 to 64 years and 8 percent for those aged 65 years and older. COPD death rates were lower in the Hispanic groups than in non-Hispanic whites; however, these rates have been increasing for Hispanics.

Women might be more susceptible than men to developing COPD when exposed to risk factors such as tobacco smoke. The beneficial effects of stopping smoking on the rate of lung function decline may be greater for women than men.

Primary care physicians are in a key position to provide optimal care to patients with COPD and to provide counseling during clinical or health center visits to patients who smoke. Effective tests are available to screen patients for COPD, and primary care physicians need to be trained in the latest methods to detect and treat the disease.

OBSTRUCTIVE SLEEP APNEA

Some 18 million persons in the United States were estimated to have Obstructive Sleep Apnea (OSA). OSA affects all races, ages, and socioeconomic and ethnic groups. Because OSA causes serious disturbances in normal sleep patterns, patients experience excessive daytime sleepiness and impaired performance. Common consequences of OSA range from personality changes and sexual dysfunction to falling asleep at work or while driving.

OSA symptoms include many repeated involuntary breathing pauses during sleep. The breathing pauses often are accompanied by choking sensations that may wake the patient. Other symptoms include intermittent snoring, awakening from sleep (poor sleep), early morning headaches, and excessive daytime sleepiness.

OSA can increase the seriousness of other lung diseases that decrease airflow, such as asthma and COPD. Cardiovascular deaths alone due to OSA have been estimated at 38,000 a year. Individuals with OSA often do not recognize reductions in alertness, diminished productivity, and discord in interpersonal relationships as part of the syndrome. Persons affected by OSA, for example, are seven times more likely to be involved in multiple vehicular crashes. In children, OSA can disrupt sleep. OSA also may cause daytime behavioral problems that affect workplace performance and affect their learning ability in school.

Infants with siblings or parents who have OSA inherit an increased risk of sudden infant death syndrome (SIDS). This tragic sleep-related breathing disorder takes the lives of more infants than all other causes combined.

OSA is prevalent particularly in men over age 50 years and in postmenopausal women, when hormonal changes appear to increase risk. The risk of OSA also is increased in certain racial and ethnic groups. Among young African Americans, the likelihood of experiencing OSA symptoms is twice that of young whites. Nearly 50 percent of OSA patients have high blood pressure.

A major factor in the pervasiveness of OSA's effects on health and society has been the failure to educate Americans—and especially health care practitioners— about the disorder. A wide range of behavioral, mechanical, and surgical treatments can be used to manage OSA symptoms. Providing persons at risk with culturally and linguistically appropriate information about OSA could enable them to prevent or lessen the effects of OSA. Improved awareness of OSA symptoms represents a major public health challenge.

Primary care providers are an important barometer of OSA awareness because they are a first stop for patients who are seeking appropriate diagnosis and treatment. However, only 79 cases of sleep disorder were diagnosed in a sample of 10 million patient records. In 1990s about a third of the medical schools in the United States offered no training in sleep medicine, and another third provided less than 2 hours on average for all sleep topics. In the absence of strong educational models for physicians, the risk remains high that OSA will be misdiagnosed and mismanaged.

8

An Aging Population

The older population (65+) numbered 43.1 million in 2012, an increase of 7.6 million or 21% since 2002, according to the Department of Health and Human Services Administration for Community Living. They represent 12.9 percent of the U.S. population, about one in every eight Americans.

By 2030, there will be about 72.1 million older persons, more than twice their number in 2000. People 65+ represented 12.4% of the population in the year 2000 but are expected to grow to be 19% of the population by 2030.

A PROFILE

- The older population (65+) numbered 43.1 million in 2012, an increase of 7.6 million or 21% since 2002.
- The number of Americans aged 45-64 – who will reach 65 over the next two decades – increased by 24% between 2002 and 2012.
- About one in every seven, or 13.7%, of the population is an older American.
- Persons reaching age 65 have an average life expectancy of an additional 19.2 years (20.4 years for females and 17.8 years for males).
- Older women outnumber older men at 24.3 million older women to 18.8 million older men.
- In 2012, 21.0% of persons 65+ were members of racial or ethnic minority populations--9% were African-Americans (not Hispanic), 4% were Asian or Pacific Islander (not Hispanic), .5% were Native American (not Hispanic), and 0.7% of persons 65+ identified

themselves as being of two or more races. Persons of Hispanic origin (who may be of any race) represented 7% of the older population.

• Older men were much more likely to be married than older women--71% of men vs. 45% of women (Figure 2). In 2013, 36% older women were widows.

• About 28% (12.1 million) of noninstitutionalized older persons live alone (8.4 million women, 3.7 million men).

• Almost half of older women (45%) age 75+ live alone.

• In 2012, about 518,000 grandparents aged 65 or more had the primary responsibility for their grandchildren who lived with them.

• The population 65 and over has increased from 35.5 million in 2002 to 43.1 million in 2012 (a 21% increase) and is projected to increase to 79.7 million in 2040.

• The 85+ population is projected to increase from 5.9 million in 2012 to 14.1 million in 2040.

• Racial and ethnic minority populations have increased from 6.1 million in 2002 (17% of the elderly population) to 8.9 million in 2012 (21% of the elderly) and are projected to increase to 20.2 million in 2030 (28% of the elderly).

• The median income of older persons in 2012 was $27,612 for males and $16,040 for females. Median money income (after adjusting for inflation) of all households headed by older people rose by .1% (not statistically significant) from 2011 to 2012. Households containing families headed by persons 65+ reported a median income in 2012 of $48,957.

• The major sources of income as reported by older persons in 2011 were Social Security (reported by 86% of older persons), income from assets (reported by 52%), private pensions (reported by 27%), government employee pensions (reported by 15%), and earnings (reported by 28%).

• Social Security constituted 90% or more of the income received by 35% of beneficiaries in 2011 (22% of married couples and 45% of non-married beneficiaries).

• Over 3.9 million elderly persons (9.1%) were below the poverty level in 2012. This poverty rate is statistically different from the poverty rate in 2011 (8.7%). In 2011, the U.S. Census Bureau also released a new Supplemental Poverty Measure (SPM) which takes into account regional variations in the livings costs, non-cash benefits received, and non-discretionary expenditures but does not replace the official poverty measure. In 2012, the SPM shows a poverty level for older persons of 14.8% (more than 5 percentage points higher than the official rate of 9.1%). This increase is mainly due to including medical out-of-pocket expenses in the poverty calculations.

Principal sources of data for the Profile are the U.S. Census Bureau, the National Center for Health Statistics, and the Bureau of Labor Statistics.

The older population—persons 65 years or older—numbered 43.1 million in 2012 (the most recent year for which data are available). They represented 13.7% of the U.S. population, about one in every seven Americans. The number of older Americans increased by 7.6 million or 21% since 2002, compared to an increase of 7% for the under-65 population. However, the number of Americans aged 45-64 – who will reach 65 over the next two decades – increased by 24% between 2002 and 2012.

In 2012, there were 24.3 million older women and 18.8 million older men, or a sex ratio of 129 women for every 100 men. At age 85 and over, this ratio increases to 200 women for every 100 men.

Since 1900, the percentage of Americans 65+ has more than tripled (from 4.1% in 1900 to 13.7% in 2012), and the number has increased over thirteen times (from 3.1 million to 43.1 million). The older population itself is increasingly older. In 2012, the 65-74 age group (24 million) was more than 10 times larger than in 1900; the 75-84 group (13.3 million) was 17 times larger and the 85+ group (5.9 million) was 48 times larger.

In 2011, persons reaching age 65 had an average life expectancy of an additional 19.2 years (20.4 years for females and 17.8 years for males). A child born in 2011 could expect to live 78.7 years, about 30 years longer than a child born in 1900. Much of this increase occurred because of reduced death rates for children and young adults. However, the period of 1990-2007 also has seen reduced death rates for the population aged 65-84, especially for men – by 41.6% for men aged 65-74 and by 29.5% for men aged 75-84. Life expectancy at age 65 increased by only 2.5 years between 1900 and 1960, but has increased by 4.2 years from 1960 to 2007. Nonetheless, some research has raised concerns about future increases in life expectancy in the US compared to other high-income countries, primarily due to past smoking and current obesity levels, especially for women age 50 and over.

About 3.6 million persons celebrated their 65th birthday in 2012. Census estimates showed an annual net increase between 2011 and 2012 of 1.8 million in the number of persons 65 and over.

Between 1980 and 2012, the centenarian population experienced a larger percentage increase than did the total population. There were 61,985 persons aged 100 or more in 2012 (0.14% of the total 65+ population). This is a 93% increase from the 1980 figure of 32,194.

FUTURE GROWTH

The older population will continue to grow significantly in the future. This growth slowed somewhat during the 1990's because of the relatively small number of babies born during the Great Depression of the 1930's. But the older population is beginning to burgeon as the "baby boom" generation begins to reach age 65.

The population 65 and over has increased from 35.5 million in 2002 to 43.1 million in 2012 (a 21% increase) and is projected to more than double to 92 million in 2060. By 2040, there will be about 79.7 million older persons, over twice their number in 2000. People 65+ represented 13.7% of the population in the year 2012 but are expected to grow to be 21% of the population by 2040. The 85+ population is projected to triple from 5.9 million in 2012 to 14.1 million in 2040.

Racial and ethnic minority populations have increased from 6.1 million in 2002 (17% of the elderly population) to 8.9 million in 2012 (21% of the elderly) and are projected to increase to 20.2 million in 2030 (28% of the elderly). Between 2012 and 2030, the white (not Hispanic) population 65+ is projected to increase by 54% compared with 126% for older racial and ethnic minority populations, including Hispanics (155%), African-Americans (not Hispanic) (104%), American Indian and Native Alaskans (not Hispanic) (116%), and Asians (not Hispanic) (119%).

CHARACTERISTICS OF THE AGING POPULATION

Marital Status

Marital Status In 2013, older men were much more likely to be married than older women—71% of men, 45% of women (Figure 2). Widows accounted for 36% of all older women in 2013. There were more than three times as many widows (8.7 million) as widowers (2.3 million).

Divorced and separated (including married/spouse absent) older persons represented only 13% of all older persons in 2013. However, this percentage has increased since 1980, when approximately 5.3% of the older population were divorced or separated/spouse absent.

Marital Status In 2013, older men were much more likely to be married than older women—71% of men, 45% of women (Figure 2). Widows accounted for 36% of all older women in 2013. There were more than three times as many widows (8.7 million) as widowers (2.3 million).

Divorced and separated (including married/spouse absent) older persons represented only 13% of all older persons in 2013. However, this percentage has increased since 1980, when approximately 5.3% of the older population were divorced or separated/spouse absent.

Living Arrangements

Over half (57%) the older noninstitutionalized persons lived with their spouse in 2013. Approximately 13.8 million or 71% of older men, and 10.7 million or 45% of older women, lived with their spouse (Figure 3). The proportion living with their spouse decreased with age, especially for women. Only 32% of women 75+ years old lived with a spouse.

About 28% (12.1 million) of all noninstitutionalized older persons in 2013 lived alone (8.4 million women, 3.7 million men). They represented 35% of older women and 19% of older men. The proportion living alone increases with advanced age. Among women aged 75 and over, for example, almost half (45%) lived alone.

In 2012, a total of about 2.1 million older people lived in a household with a grandchild present. About 518,000 of these grandparents over 65 years old were the persons with primary responsibility for their grandchildren who lived with them.

A relatively small number (1.5 million) and percentage (3.5%) of the 65+ population in 2012 lived in institutional settings such as nursing homes (1.2 million). However, the percentage increases dramatically with age, ranging (in 2012) from 1% for persons 65-74 years to 3% for persons 75-84 years and 10% for persons 85+. In addition, in 2009, approximately 2.7% of the elderly lived in senior housing with at least one supportive service available to their residents.

Racial and Ethnic Composition

In 2012, 21.0% of persons 65+ were members of racial or ethnic minority populations--9% were African- Americans (not Hispanic), 4% were Asian or Pacific Islander (not Hispanic), .5% were Native American (not Hispanic), .1% were Native Hawaiian/Pacific Islander, (not Hispanic), and 0.7% of persons 65+ identified themselves as being of two or more races. Persons of Hispanic origin (who may be of any race) represented 7% of the older population.

Only 7.7% of all the people who were members of racial and ethnic minority populations were 65+ in 2012 (9.5% of African-Americans (not Hispanic), 5.9% of Hispanics, 10.3% of Asians, 7% of Native Hawaiian and Other Pacific Islanders (not Hispanic), 8.9% of American Indian and Native Alaskans (not Hispanic)) compared with 17.3% of non-Hispanic whites.

Geographic Distribution

The proportion of older persons in the population varies considerably by state with some states experiencing much greater growth in their older populations. In 2012, over half (59%) of persons 65+ lived in 12 states: California (4.6 million); Florida (3.5 million); Texas (2.8 million); New York (2.8 million); Pennsylvania (2.0 million); and Ohio, Illinois, Michigan, North Carolina, New Jersey, Virginia, and Georgia each had well over 1 million.

Persons 65+ constituted approximately 15% or more of the total population in 11 states in 2012: Florida (18.2%); Maine (17.0%); West Virginia (16.8%); Pennsylvania (16.0%); Montana (15.7%); Vermont (15.7%); Delaware (15.3%); Iowa (15.3%); Hawaii (15.1%); Rhode Island (15.1%); and Arkansas (15.0%). In 14 states, the 65+ population increased by 30% or more between 2002 and 2012: Alaska (58.9%), Nevada (49.3%), Colorado (41.7%), Georgia (40.1%), Arizona (39.6%); Idaho (39.1%), South Carolina (39.1%), Utah (36.6%), North Carolina (34.6%), Washington (33.9%); New Mexico (33.6%); Delaware (33.6%); Texas (33.2%); and Virginia (30.2%). The 17 jurisdictions with poverty rates at or over 10% for elderly during 2012 were: Mississippi (15.1%), Louisiana (12.6%), Kentucky (12.3%), District of Columbia (11.9%), New Mexico (11.9%), Texas (11.6%), New York (11.4%), Georgia (11.2%), Alabama (11.1%), Arkansas (10.9%), North Dakota (10.6%), California (10.4%), Florida (10.2%), South Carolina (10.1%), North Carolina (10.0%), South Dakota (10.0%), and Tennessee (10%).

Most persons 65+ lived in metropolitan areas in 2012 (81%). About 66% of these older persons lived outside principal cities and 34% lived inside principal cities. Also, 19% of older persons lived outside of metropolitan areas.

The elderly are less likely to change residence than other age groups. From 2012 to 2013, only 4% of older persons moved as opposed to 13% of the under 65 population. Most older movers (57%) stayed in the same county and 81% remained in the same state. Only 19% of the movers moved from out-of-state or abroad.

Income

The median income of older persons in 2012 was $27,612 for males and $16,040 for females. From 2011 to 2012, median money income (after adjusting for inflation) of all households headed by older people rose .1% but this was not statistically significant. Households containing families headed by persons 65+ reported a median income in 2012 of $48,957 ($50,701 for non-Hispanic Whites, $33,913 for Hispanics, $40,348 for African-Americans, and $56,378 for Asians). About 5% of family households with an elderly householder had incomes less than $15,000 and 67% had incomes of $35,000 or more.

For all older persons reporting income in 2012 (41.8 million), 17% reported less than $10,000 and 41% reported $25,000 or more. The median income reported was $20,380. The major sources of income as reported by older persons in 2011 were Social Security (reported by 86% of older persons), income from assets (reported by 52%), private pensions (reported by 27%), government employee pensions (reported by 15%), and earnings (reported by 28%). In 2011, Social Security benefits accounted for 36% of the aggregate income of the older population. The bulk of the remainder consisted of earnings (32%), asset income (11%), and pensions (18%). Social Security constituted 90% or more of the income received by 35% of beneficiaries (22% of married couples and 45% of non-married beneficiaries).

Poverty

Over 3.9 million elderly persons (9.1%) were below the poverty level in 2012. This poverty rate is statistically different from the poverty rate in 2011 (8.7%). Another 2.4 million or 5.5% of the elderly were classified as "near-poor" (income between the poverty level and 125% of this level). Just over 2.3 million older Whites (not Hispanic) (6.8%) were poor in 2012, compared to 18.2% of elderly African-Americans, 12.3% of Asians, and 20.6% of elderly Hispanics. Higher than average poverty rates were found in 2012 for older persons who lived inside principal cities (12.5%) and in the South (10.2%). Older women had a higher poverty rate (11%) than older men (6.6%) in 2012. Older persons living alone were much more likely to be poor (16.8%) than were older persons living with families (5.4%). The highest poverty rates were experienced among older Hispanic women (41.6%) who lived alone and also by older Black women (33%) who lived alone. In 2011, the U.S. Census Bureau released a new Supplemental Poverty Measure (SPM). The SPM methodology shows a significantly higher number of older persons below poverty than is shown by the official poverty measure. For persons 65 and older this poverty measure shows a poverty level of 14.8% in 2012 (more than 5 percentage points higher than the official rate of 9.1%). Unlike the official poverty rate, the SPM takes into account regional variations in the cost of housing etc. and, even more significantly, the impact of both non-cash benefits received (e.g., SNAP/food stamps, low income tax credits, WIC, etc.) and non-discretionary expenditures including medical out-of-pocket (MOOP) expenses. For persons 65 and over, MOOP was the major source of the significant differences between these measures. Bear in mind that the SPM does not replace the official poverty measure.

Housing

Of the 25.1 million households headed by older persons in 2011, 81% were owners and 19% were renters. The median family income of older homeowners was $32,900. The median family income of older renters was $16,200. In 2011, almost 50% of older householders spent more than one-fourth of their income on housing costs - 43% for owners and 71% for renters - as compared to 50% of all householders. For older homeowners in 2011, the median construction year was 1970 compared with 1976 for all homeowners. Among the homes owned by people age 65 and older, 3.3% had physical problems. In 2011, the median value of homes owned by older persons was $150,000 (with a median purchase price of $55,000) compared to a median home value of $160,000 for all homeowners. About 65% of older homeowners in 2011 owned their homes free and clear.

Employment

In 2013, 8.1 million (18.7 %) Americans age 65 and over were in the labor force (working or actively seeking work), including 4.5 million men (23.5%) and 3.6 million women (14.9%). They constituted 5% of the U.S. labor force. About 5.4% were unemployed. Labor force participation of men 65+ decreased steadily from two thirds in 1900 to 15.8% in 1985; then stayed at 16%-18% until 2002; and has been increasing since then to over 20%. The participation rate for women 65+ rose slightly from 1 of 12 in 1900 to 10.8% in 1956, fell to 7.3% in 1985, was around 7%-9% from 1986 – 2002. However, beginning in 2000, labor force participation of older women has been gradually rising to the 2013 level. This increase is especially noticeable among the population aged 65-69.

Education

The educational level of the older population is increasing. Between 1970 and 2013, the percentage of older persons who had completed high school rose from 28% to 83%. About 25% in 2013 had a bachelor's degree or higher. The percentage who had completed high school varied considerably by race and ethnic origin in 2013: 87% of Whites (not Hispanic), 76% of Asians, 71% of African-Americans, 60% of American Indian/Alaska Natives (in 2012), and 51% of Hispanics. The increase in educational levels is also evident within these groups. In 1970, only 30% of older Whites and 9% of older African-Americans were high school graduates.

HEALTH AND HEALTH CARE

In 2010-2012, 42% of noninstitutionalized people age 65 and over assessed their health as excellent or very good (compared to 55% for persons aged 45-64 years). There was little difference between the sexes on this measure, but older African-Americans (not Hispanic) (26%), older American Indians/Alaska Natives (31%), older Asians (34%), and older Hispanics (31%) were less likely to rate their health as excellent or very good than were older Whites (not Hispanic) (46%).

Most older persons have at least one chronic condition and many have multiple conditions. In 2010-2012, the most frequently occurring conditions among older persons were: diagnosed arthritis (50%), all types of heart disease (30%), any cancer (24%), diagnosed diabetes (20% in 2007-2010), and hypertension (high blood pressure or taking antihypertensive medication) (72 percent in 2007-2010). In January-June 2013, 69% of people age 65 and over reported that they received an influenza vaccination during the past 12 months and 61% reported that they had ever received a pneumococcal vaccination. About 27% (of persons 60+) reported height/weight combinations that placed them among the obese.

Slightly over 42% of persons aged 65-74 and 29% of persons 75+ reported that they engaged in regular leisure-time physical activity. Only 8% reported that they are current smokers and 7% reported excessive alcohol consumption. Only 2% reported that they had experienced psychological distress during the past 30 days. In 2009-2010, about 13.8 million persons aged 65 and older were discharged from short stay hospitals. This is a rate of 3,436.1 for every 10,000 persons aged 65+ which is about three times the comparable rate for persons of all ages (which was 1,125.1 per 10,000). The average length of stay for persons aged 65-74 5.4 days; for ages 75-84 it was 5.7 days; and for ages 85 and over it was 5.6 days. The comparable rate for persons of all ages was 4.8 days.

The average length of stay for older people has decreased by 5 days since 1980. Older persons averaged more office visits with doctors in 2012. Among people age 75 and over, 23 percent had 10 or more visits to a doctor or other health care professional in the past 12 months compared to 14 percent among people age 45 to 64. In January-June 2013, 96% of older persons reported that they did have a usual place to go for medical care and only 2.3% said that they failed to obtain needed medical care during the previous 12 months due to financial barriers.

In 2012 older consumers averaged out-of-pocket health care expenditures of $5,118, an increase of 43% since 2002. In contrast, the total population spent considerably less, averaging $3,556 in out-of-pocket costs. Older Americans spent 12.7% of their total expenditures on health, almost twice the proportion spent by all consumers (6.9%). Health costs incurred on average by older consumers in 2012 consisted of $3,186 (62%) for insurance, $935 (18%) for medical services, $798 (16%) for drugs, and $200 (4.0%) for medical supplies.

HEALTH INSURANCE COVERAGE

In 2012, almost all (93%) non-institutionalized persons 65+ were covered by Medicare. Medicare covers mostly acute care services and requires beneficiaries to pay part of the cost, leaving about half of health spending to be covered by other sources. About 56% had some type of private health insurance. Almost 9% had military-based health insurance and 8% of the non-institutionalized elderly were covered by Medicaid. Less than 2% did not have coverage of some kind. About 86% of non-institutionalized Medicare beneficiaries in 2009 had some type of supplementary coverage. Among Medicare beneficiaries residing in nursing homes in 2010, almost half (49%) were covered by Medicaid.

Some type of disability (i.e., difficulty in hearing, vision, cognition, ambulation, self-care, or independent living) was reported by 36% of people age 65 and over in 2012. The percentages for individual disabilities ranged from almost one quarter (23 percent) having an ambulatory disability to 7 percent having a vision difficulty. Some of these disabilities may be relatively minor but others cause people to require assistance to meet important personal needs. There is a strong relationship between disability status and reported health status. Presence of a severe disability is also associated with lower income levels and educational attainment.

Using limitations in activities of daily living (ADLs) and instrumental activities of daily living (IADLs) to measure disability, in 2010, 28% of community-resident Medicare beneficiaries age 65+ reported difficulty in performing one or more ADLs and an additional 12% reported difficulty with one or more IADLs. By contrast, 92% of institutionalized Medicare beneficiaries had difficulties with one or more ADLs and 76% of them had difficulty with three or more ADLs. [ADLs include bathing, dressing, eating, and getting around the house. IADLs include preparing meals, shopping, managing money, using the telephone, doing housework, and taking medication.] Limitations in activities because of chronic conditions increase with age. Except where noted, the figures above are taken from surveys of the noninstitutionalized elderly. Although nursing homes are being increasingly used for short-stay post-acute care, about 1.3 million elderly are in nursing homes (more than half are age 85 and over). These individuals often need care with their ADLs and/or have severe cognitive impairment due to Alzheimer's disease or other dementias.

MEDICARE

Medicare, the federal health insurance program for 54 million people ages 65 and over and people with permanent disabilities, helps to pay for hospital and physician visits, prescription drugs, and other acute and post-acute services. In 2013, spending on Medicare accounted for 14% of the federal budget. Medicare also plays a major role in the health care system, accounting for 20% of total national health spending in 2012, 27% of spending on hospital care, and 23% of spending on physician services.

Medicare benefit payments totaled $583 billion in 2013; roughly one-fourth was for hospital inpatient services, 12% for physician services, and 11% for the Part D drug benefit. Another one-fourth of benefit spending was for Medicare Advantage private health plans covering all Part A and B benefits; in 2014, 30% of Medicare beneficiaries are enrolled in Medicare Advantage plans.

Both in the aggregate and on a per capita basis, Medicare spending growth has slowed in recent years and is expected to grow at a slower rate in the future than in the past—and even slower than was projected just a few years ago. And in a break from the historical pattern, net Medicare spending is projected to be a roughly constant share of the federal budget and the nation's economy in the coming decade.

On a historical basis, Medicare spending per enrollee grew at an average annual rate of 7.7% between 1969 and 2012, slower than the 9.2% average annual growth rate in private health insurance spending per enrollee (this comparison includes benefits commonly covered by Medicare and private health insurance over this period, including hospital services, physician and clinical services, and other professional services, and durable medical products).

More recently, total and per capita Medicare spending have grown more slowly each year since 2010. Based on a comparison of CBO's August 2010 and April 2014 baselines, Medicare spending in 2014 will be about $1,000 lower per person than was expected in 2010, soon after passage of the 2010 Affordable Care Act (ACA).

Medicare spending projections in CBO's August 2010 and subsequent baselines take into account the anticipated effects of the ACA, along with other factors that are expected to affect future Medicare spending. The ACA included reductions in Medicare payments to plans and providers and introduced delivery system reforms that aimed to improve efficiency and quality of patient care and reduce costs, including accountable care organizations (ACOs), medical homes, bundled payments, and value-based purchasing initiatives. The law also increased the Medicare Part A payroll tax rate on earnings for higher-income people and increased Part B and Part D premiums for higher-income beneficiaries. In addition, the Budget Control Act of 2011 lowered Medicare spending through sequestration that reduced payments to providers and plans by 2% beginning in 2013.

Future Trends in Medicare Spending

Looking ahead, net Medicare outlays (that is, Medicare spending minus income from premiums and other offsetting receipts) are projected to increase by two-thirds from $512 billion in 2014 to $858 billion in 2024—an average annual growth rate of 5.3% in the aggregate—due to growth in the Medicare population and increases in health care costs. These estimates do not take into account additional spending that is likely to occur to avoid reductions in physician fees scheduled under current law. The growth in health spending, which affects all payers, is influenced by increasing volume and use of services, new technologies, and increasing prices.

Yet despite annual growth in outlays, net Medicare spending is projected to be a roughly constant share of the federal budget and the nation's economy in the coming decade. Medicare's share of the federal budget is projected to be 14.5% in both 2014 and 2024 (varying slightly between these years), while Medicare spending as a share of GDP is projected to be 3.0% in 2014 and 3.2% in 2024. On a per capita basis, Medicare spending is projected to grow at a slower rate between 2013 and 2022 than it did between 2000 and 2012 (4.0% vs. 6.1%). Medicare spending also is projected to grow more slowly than private health insurance spending on a per capita basis in the coming years. According to CBO, in the coming decade (2015-2024), the rate of Medicare per capita spending growth will be roughly in line with growth in GDP per capita, while private health insurance premiums are expected to grow 2 percentage points faster.

Over the longer term, however, both CBO and the Medicare Actuaries expect Medicare spending to begin to rise more rapidly due to a number of factors, including the aging of the population, an increase in service use associated with greater severity of illness, and faster growth in health care costs than growth in the economy on a per capita basis. According to CBO's most recent long-term projections, net Medicare spending will grow from 3.0% of GDP in 2014 to 3.8% of GDP in 2030, 4.7% in 2040, and 5.5% in 2050. Through 2039, CBO projects that the aging of the population will account for a larger share of spending growth on the nation's major health care programs (Medicare, Medicaid, and subsidies for ACA Marketplace coverage) than either "excess" health care spending growth or expansion of Medicaid and Marketplace subsidies.

How Is Medicare Financed?

Medicare is funded primarily from three sources: general revenues (41%), payroll tax contributions (3%), and beneficiary premiums (13%).

Part A (the Hospital Insurance program) is financed primarily through a 2.9% tax on earnings paid by employers and employees (1.45% each) (accounting for 88% of Part A revenue). Higher-income taxpayers (more than $200,000/individual and $250,000/couple) pay a higher payroll tax on earnings (2.35%).

Part B (the Supplementary Medical Insurance program) is financed through general revenues (73%), beneficiary premiums (25%), and interest and other sources (2%). Beneficiaries with annual incomes over $85,000/individual or $170,000/couple pay a higher, income-related Part B premium reflecting a larger share of total Part B spending, ranging from 35% to 80%; the ACA froze the income thresholds through 2019, which is expected to increase the share of beneficiaries paying the higher Part B premium.

Part D is financed through general revenues (73%), beneficiary premiums (14%), and state payments for dual eligibles (13%). Similar to Part B, enrollees with higher incomes pay a larger share of the cost of Part D coverage.

The Medicare Advantage program (Part C) is not separately financed. Medicare Advantage plans such as HMOs and PPOs cover all Part A, Part B, and (typically) Part D benefits. Beneficiaries enrolled in Medicare Advantage plans typically pay monthly premiums for additional benefits covered by their plan in addition to the Part B premium.

Solvency of the Medicare Hospital Insurance Trust Fund

The solvency of the Medicare Hospital Insurance trust fund, out of which Part A benefits are paid, is a common way of measuring Medicare's financial status. Solvency is measured by the level of assets in the Part A trust fund. In years when annual income to the trust fund exceeds benefits spending, the asset level increases, and when annual spending exceeds income, the asset level decreases. When spending exceeds income and the assets are fully depleted, Medicare will not have sufficient funds to pay all Part A benefits.

Each year, the Medicare Trustees provide an estimate of the year when the asset level is projected to be fully depleted. Because of slower growth in Medicare spending in recent years, the solvency of the trust fund has been extended. In 2014, the Trustees project that the Part A trust fund will be depleted in 2030, four years later than was projected in the 2013 report and six years later than was projected in the 2012 report.

Part A Trust Fund solvency is affected by growth in the economy, which affects revenue from payroll tax contributions, health care spending trends, and demographic trends: an increasing number of beneficiaries, especially between 2010 and 2030 when the baby boom generation reaches Medicare eligibility age, and a declining ratio of workers per beneficiary making payroll tax contributions.

Part B and Part D do not have financing challenges similar to Part A, because both are funded by beneficiary premiums and general revenues that are set annually to match expected outlays. However, future increases in spending under Part B and Part D will require increases in general revenue funding and higher premiums paid by beneficiaries.

In addition to the solvency of the Part A trust fund, Medicare's financial condition can be measured in other ways. For example, the Independent Payment Advisory Board (IPAB), which was authorized by the ACA, is required to recommend Medicare spending reductions to Congress if projected spending growth exceeds specified target levels. IPAB is required to propose spending reductions if the 5-year average growth rate in Medicare per capita spending is projected to exceed the per capita target growth rate, based on inflation (2015-2019) or growth in the economy (2020 and beyond). The ACA required the IPAB process to begin in 2013, but CBO has estimated that spending reductions will not be triggered for several years because Medicare spending growth is expected to be below the target growth rate during the next decade.

Future Outlook

Several questions remain unanswered about recent trends in Medicare spending and what they portend about future spending levels: What are the primary reasons for the recent slowdown in Medicare spending? How are delivery system reforms influencing the Medicare spending trajectory? Are the Medicare changes in the ACA having an even larger effect on spending than expected? Can the slowdown be sustained and can this be done without adversely affecting access to or quality of care?

While Medicare spending is on a slower upward trajectory now than in the past, Medicare is likely to be a focus of future policy discussions about reducing the federal budget debt, given the health care financing challenges posed by the aging of the population. A number of changes to Medicare have been proposed, including: restructuring Medicare benefits and cost sharing; eliminating "first-dollar" Medigap coverage; increasing Medicare premiums for all beneficiaries or those with relatively high incomes; raising the Medicare eligibility age; shifting Medicare from a defined benefit structure to a "premium support" system; and accelerating the ACA's delivery system reforms.

How the recent slowdown in Medicare spending growth will affect the prospects for these proposals is unclear, but it could provide an opportunity for thoughtful consideration of these and other ways to bolster the program for an aging population.

9

Alzheimer's and Dementia

Dementia is the name for a group of symptoms caused by disorders that affect the brain. It is not a specific disease. Dementia is the loss of cognitive functioning—thinking, remembering, and reasoning—and behavioral abilities to such an extent that it interferes with a person's daily life and activities.

People with dementia may not be able to think well enough to do normal activities, such as getting dressed or eating. They may lose their ability to solve problems or control their emotions. Their personalities may change. They may become agitated or see things that are not there.

Memory loss is a common symptom of dementia. However, memory loss by itself does not mean you have dementia. People with dementia have serious problems with two or more brain functions, such as memory and language. Although dementia is common in very elderly people, it is not part of normal aging.

Many different diseases can cause dementia, including Alzheimer's disease and stroke. Drugs are available to treat some of these diseases. While these drugs cannot cure dementia or repair brain damage, they may improve symptoms or slow down the disease. Alzheimer's is the most common type of dementia.

OTHER DEMENTIAS

Dementia ranges in severity from the mildest stage, when it is just beginning to affect a person's functioning, to the most severe stage, when the person must depend completely on others for basic activities of daily living.

Many conditions and diseases cause dementia. The most common cause of dementia in older people is Alzheimer's disease. Other causes include different kinds of brain changes that lead to vascular dementia, Lewy body dementia, and frontotemporal disorders.

In addition, some people have mixed dementia—a combination of two or more disorders, at least one of which is dementia. A number of combinations are possible. For example, some people have Alzheimer's disease and vascular dementia at the same time.

Other causes of dementia include Huntington's disease, Creutzfeldt-Jakob disease, head injury, and HIV. In addition, some conditions that cause dementia, such as normal pressure hydrocephalus, thyroid problems, and vitamin B deficiency, can be reversed with appropriate treatment.

Vascular dementia

Vascular dementia, considered the second most common form of dementia after Alzheimer's disease, results from injuries to the vessels supplying blood to the brain, often after a stroke or series of strokes. Vascular dementia and vascular cognitive impairment arise as a result of risk factors that similarly increase the risk for cerebrovascular disease (stroke), including atrial fibrillation, hypertension, diabetes, and high cholesterol. The symptoms of vascular dementia can be similar to those of Alzheimer's, and both conditions can occur at the same time. Symptoms of vascular dementia can begin suddenly and worsen or improve during one's lifetime.

Some types of vascular dementia include:

- Multi-infarct dementia
- Cerebral autosomal dominant arteriopathy with subcortical infarcts and leukoencephalopathy (CADASIL)
- Subcortical vascular dementia (Binswanger's disease)

Research has shown that Alzheimer's and vascular disease-associated cognitive impairment are closely intertwined. For example, a large proportion of people diagnosed with Alzheimer's also have brain damage caused by vascular disease. In addition, several studies have found that many of the major risk factors for vascular disease may also be risk factors for Alzheimer's.

The overlap between these two types of dementia may be important because medications and lifestyle changes known to help prevent vascular disease, such as controlling high blood pressure, lowering

Lewy Body Dementia

Lewy body dementia (LBD) is another common brain disorder in older people. LBD is caused by abnormal deposits of a protein called alpha-synuclein in the brain. These deposits, called Lewy bodies, can lead to problems with thinking, movement, behavior, and mood. For example, symptoms may include changes in alertness and attention, hallucinations, tremor, muscle stiffness, sleep problems, and memory loss.

The two types of LBD are:

Dementia with Lewy bodies, in which cognitive symptoms appear within a year of movement problems

Parkinson's disease dementia, in which cognitive problems develop more than a year after the onset of movement problems

Lewy body dementia can be hard to diagnose because Parkinson's disease and Alzheimer's disease cause similar symptoms. Scientists think that LBD might be related to these diseases, or that they sometimes happen together.

Frontotemporal Disorders

Frontotemporal disorders are a form of dementia caused by a family of brain diseases known as frontotemporal lobar degeneration (FTLD). These disorders are the result of damage to neurons (nerve cells) in parts of the brain called the frontal and temporal lobes. As neurons die in the frontal and temporal regions, these lobes atrophy, or shrink. Gradually, this damage causes difficulties in thinking and behaviors controlled by these parts of the brain. Many possible symptoms can result. They include strange behaviors, emotional problems, trouble communicating, or difficulty with walking and other basic movements.

Frontotemporal disorders can be grouped into three types, defined by the earliest symptoms physicians identify when they examine patients. The following conditions are frontotemporal disorders:

- Behavioral variant frontotemporal dementia (bvFTD)
- Pick's disease
- Primary progressive aphasia (PPA)
- Corticobasal syndrome
- Progressive supranuclear palsy (PSP)
- Frontotemporal dementia with parkinsonism

- Frontotemporal dementia with amyotrophic lateral sclerosis (FTD-ALS)

Mixed Dementia

Autopsy studies looking at the brains of people who had dementia suggest that a majority of those age 80 and older probably had "mixed dementia," caused by processes related to both Alzheimer's disease and vascular disease. In fact, some studies indicate that mixed vascular-degenerative dementia is the most common cause of dementia in the elderly. In a person with mixed dementia, it may not be clear exactly how many of a person's symptoms are due to Alzheimer's or another type of dementia. In one study, about 40 percent of people who were thought to have Alzheimer's were found after autopsy to also have some form of cerebrovascular disease. Several studies have found that many of the major risk factors for vascular disease also may be risk factors for Alzheimer's disease.

Researchers are still working to understand how underlying disease processes in mixed dementia influence each other. It is not clear, for example, if symptoms are likely to be worse when a person has brain changes reflecting multiple types of dementia. Nor do we know if a person with multiple dementias can benefit from treating one type, for example, when a person with Alzheimer's disease controls high blood pressure and other vascular disease risk factors.

Other conditions that cause dementia

- Creutzfeldt-Jakob disease (CJD)
- Huntington's disease
- Secondary dementias
- Head injury and chronic traumatic encephalopathy
- HIV-associated dementia (HAD)
- Reversible dementias

ALZHEIMERS' DISEASE

An estimated 5.2 million Americans had Alzheimer's disease in 2014, including approximately 200,000 individuals younger than age 65 who have younger-onset Alzheimer's. Almost two-thirds of American seniors living with Alzheimer's are women. Of the 5 million people age 65 and older with

Alzheimer's in the United States, 3.2 million are women and 1.8 million are men. The number of Americans with Alzheimer's disease and other dementias will escalate rapidly in coming years as the baby boom generation ages. By 2050, the number of people age 65 and older with Alzheimer's disease may nearly triple, from 5 million to as many as 16 million, barring the development of medical breakthroughs to prevent, slow or stop the disease.

More than 500,000 seniors die each year because they have Alzheimer's. If Alzheimer's was eliminated, half a million lives would be saved a year. Alzheimer's is officially the 6th leading cause of death in the United States and the 5th leading cause of death for those aged 65 and older. It is the fifth-leading cause of death in women, and the tenth in men. However, it may cause even more deaths than official sources recognize. It kills more than prostate cancer and breast cancer combined.

Deaths from Alzheimer's increased 68 percent between 2000 and 2010, while deaths from other major diseases decreased. Alzheimer's disease is the only cause of death among the top 10 in America that cannot be prevented, cured or even slowed.

The Global Costs

The cause of most dementia is unknown, but the final stages of this disease usually means a loss of memory, reasoning, speech, and other cognitive functions, according to HHS's National Institute on Aging. The risk of dementia increases sharply with age and, unless new strategies for prevention and management are developed, this syndrome is expected to place growing demands on health and long-term care providers as the world's population ages. Dementia prevalence estimates vary considerably internationally, in part because diagnoses and reporting systems are not standardized. The disease is not easy to diagnose, especially in its early stages. The memory problems, misunderstandings, and behavior common in the early and intermediate stages are often attributed to normal effects of aging, accepted as personality traits, or simply ignored. Many cases remain undiagnosed even in the intermediate, more serious stages. A cross-national assessment conducted by the Organization for Economic Cooperation and Development (OECD) estimated that dementia affected about 10 million people in OECD member countries around 2000, just under 7 percent of people aged 65 or older.

Alzheimer's disease (AD) is the most common form of dementia and accounted for between two-fifths and four-fifths of all dementia cases cited in the OECD report. More recent analyses have estimated the worldwide number of people living with AD/dementia at between 27 million and 36 million. The prevalence of AD and other dementias is very low at younger ages, then nearly doubles with every five years of age after age 65. In the OECD review, for example, dementia affected fewer than 3 percent of those aged 65 to 69, but almost 30 percent of those aged 85 to 89. More than one-half of women aged 90 or older had dementia in France and Germany, as did about 40 percent in the United States, and just under 30 percent in Spain.

The projected costs of caring for the growing numbers of people with dementia are daunting. The 2010 World Alzheimer Report 141 by Alzheimer's Disease International estimates that the total worldwide cost of dementia exceeded US$600 billion in 2010, including informal care provided by family and others, social care provided by community care professionals, and direct costs of medical care. Family members often play a key caregiving role, especially in the initial stages of what is typically a slow decline. Ten years ago, U.S. researchers estimated that the annual cost of informal caregiving for dementia in the United States was US$18 billion.

The complexity of the disease and the wide variety of living arrangements can be difficult for people and families dealing with dementia, and countries must cope with the mounting financial and social impact. The challenge is even greater in the less developed world, where an estimated two-thirds or more of dementia sufferers live but where few coping resources are available. Projections by Alzheimer's Disease International suggest that 115 million people worldwide will be living with AD/dementia in 2050, with a markedly increasing proportion of this total in less developed countries. Global efforts are underway to understand and find cures or ways of preventing such age-related diseases as Alzheimer's.

Alzheimer's disease is the most expensive condition in the U.S. In 2014, the direct costs to American society of caring for those with Alzheimer's will total an estimated $214 billion, including $150 billion in costs to Medicare and Medicaid. Despite these staggering figures, Alzheimer's will cost an estimated $1.2 trillion (in today's dollars) in 2050.

Nearly one in every five dollars spent by Medicare is on people with Alzheimer's or another dementia. The average per-person Medicare spending for those with Alzheimer's and other dementias is three times higher than for those without these conditions. The average per-person Medicaid spending for seniors with Alzheimer's and other dementias is 19 times higher than average per-person Medicaid spending for all other seniors.

The financial toll of Alzheimer's on families rivals the costs to Medicaid. Total Medicaid spending for people with Alzheimer's disease is $37 billion and out-of-pocket spending for individuals with Alzheimer's and other dementias is estimated at $36 billion.

Risk Factors

Several factors determine the risk of developing dementia, including age and family history. Other factors affect the management of dementia by families, communities, and the health care system.

Aging is a well-known risk factor for Alzheimer's disease and other types of dementias. Among adults aged 65 years and older, the prevalence of Alzheimer's disease doubles every 5 years.

People with a family history of Alzheimer's disease are generally considered to be at greater risk of developing the disease. Researchers have identified 3 genes that are linked to early-onset Alzheimer's disease. Until recently, only 1 gene had been identified that increases the risk of late-onset Alzheimer's disease. However, during 2009 and 2010, international teams studying the genetics of Alzheimer's disease have identified and confirmed 3 new genes that are associated with increased risk of late-onset Alzheimer's disease.

Many individuals with Alzheimer's disease or other dementias are undiagnosed. Primary care providers do not routinely test for Alzheimer's disease. Alzheimer's disease and other dementias are more often undiagnosed in rural and minority populations than in urban or white populations.

Some chronic conditions are common in people with Alzheimer's disease and other dementias. Dementias can greatly complicate the medical management of these conditions; this increases the need for coordination of care among different specialists.

Some studies suggest that the rate of Alzheimer's is higher in certain racial or ethnic groups, such as African Americans, and scientists are exploring possible explanations.

People with specific medical histories are at greater risk of Alzheimer's, including people with:

- Down Syndrome and other intellectual and developmental disorders

- Repeated concussions (falls, sports injuries, and car accidents are common causes of concussions and TBI)
- Traumatic brain injury (TBI and mild TBI)

Being at higher risk for Alzheimer's disease does not necessarily mean that you will develop the disease. Scientists continue to explore factors that may increase your chances of having Alzheimer's and, equally important, what may protect people from developing the disease.

Lack of diagnosis seriously reduces a person's access to available treatments and valuable information. Active medical management, information and support, and coordination of medical and community services have been shown to improve quality and outcomes of care for people with dementia.

Women and Alzheimer's

Women are at the epicenter of the Alzheimer's crisis. A woman's estimated lifetime risk of developing Alzheimer's at age 65 is 1 in 6, compared with nearly 1 in 11 for a man. As real a concern as breast cancer is to women's health, women in their 60s are about twice as likely to develop Alzheimer's during the rest of their lives as they are to develop breast cancer.

Not only are women more likely to have Alzheimer's, they are also more likely to be caregivers of those with Alzheimer's. More than 3 in 5 unpaid Alzheimer's caregivers are women – and there are 2.5 more women than men who provide 24-hour care for someone with Alzheimer's.

Symptoms

Each person's experience with Alzheimer's disease or dementia is different. Even so, some symptoms are common and usually move through predictable stages, from mild to more severe, over the course of several years. The symptoms of Alzheimer's disease include loss of memory, trouble finding words, general disorientation, difficulty making judgments, as well as changes in behavior and personality.

Memory loss or confusion can be caused by other problems, too. Sometimes these same symptoms are caused by an easily treatable issue, such as reaction to a medicine taken for a different health problem, or even a vitamin deficiency. It's important to get the right diagnosis so treatment can target the right problem.

Diagnosing Alzheimer's

Getting a clear diagnosis can help you get started on planning ahead for the care and support you might need. The earlier you detect Alzheimer's, the better chance you have of treatments possibly delaying certain symptoms. Early diagnosis also allows families to better plan for the course of the disease.

When someone tells a doctor about memory problems, the doctor may check their overall health, review medicines they take, and conduct or order tests that check memory, problem solving, counting, and language skills. Sometimes, a brain scan (a CT, MRI, or other tests) might help determine whether memory complaints are caused by another condition, or Alzheimer's disease.

If a primary care doctor suspects possible Alzheimer's, he or she may refer you to a specialist who can provide a detailed diagnosis, or you may decide to go to a specialist on your own. You can find specialists through memory clinics and centers, or through local organizations or referral services.

Specialists include:

- Geriatricians manage health care in older adults. They know how the body changes as it ages and whether symptoms indicate a serious problem.
- Geriatric psychiatrists specialize in the mental and emotional health of older adults and can assess memory and thinking problems.
- Neurologists specialize in the health of the brain and central nervous system, and can conduct and review brain scans (including CTs and MRIs, as well as other tests).
- Neuropsychologists can conduct tests of memory and thinking.
- Memory clinics and centers have teams of specialists who work together to diagnose the problem. Tests often are done at the clinic or center, which can speed up diagnosis.

Alzheimer's Stages and Changes

A person with Alzheimer's will change over time, and understanding these changes can help you plan ahead. People with early stage Alzheimer's can usually take part in care decisions. Experts suggest talking about worries, concerns, and frustrations with family and friends instead of trying to figure everything out on your own. Work together to find ways to maintain independence. Take time to make financial, legal, and health care plans at this stage, before the disease progresses.

As the disease progresses, memory loss and changes in behavior and mood become more severe to the point where constant attention is necessary. At the same time, people with Alzheimer's may still enjoy normal activities.

Late stage Alzheimer's requires around-the-clock care and may require a move to a residential care facility. This stage can last anywhere from a few weeks to years.

How does Alzheimer's affect the brain?

In Alzheimer's, brain cells called neurons gradually stop working, lose connections with other neurons, and eventually die. Abnormal amounts of proteins also form plaques and tangles – major hallmarks of the disease – but we do not yet know why this happens. Over time, the brain shrinks and a person with Alzheimer's can no longer remember, think, or take part in daily activities without help.

Mild Cognitive Impairment

As some people grow older, they have more memory problems than other people their age. This condition is called Mild Cognitive Impairment (MCI). People with MCI have mild problems with thinking and memory that do not generally interfere with everyday activities. They are often aware of the forgetfulness. People with MCI can progress to Alzheimer's disease over time, but not everyone with MCI develops dementia.

Alzheimer's and Down Syndrome

Alzheimer's disease occurs three to five times more often among people with Down syndrome than the general population. People with Down syndrome are also more likely to develop Alzheimer's disease at a younger age than other adults.

As with all adults, advancing age also increases the chances that a person with Down syndrome will develop Alzheimer's disease. Estimates vary, but it is reasonable to conclude that 25 percent or more of people with Down syndrome who are older than 35 show clinical signs and symptoms of Alzheimer's-type dementia. However, it is important to note that not everyone with Down syndrome develops Alzheimer's symptoms.

Treatment

Though there is no cure for Alzheimer's, there are treatments and actions you can take to better manage life with the disease. At each stage of the disease, there are medical and care-related options that need to be considered, as well as safety issues.

Medical Treatment

There is no cure for Alzheimer's, but there are medicines that may improve quality of living and delay some symptoms. Counseling and other therapies may also be recommended.

Currently there are 4 drugs approved by the U. S. Food and Drug Administration (FDA) to treat the symptoms of the disease for some time, but they cannot stop the disease itself. Not every drug will be helpful for every person with dementia.

Treating the symptoms of Alzheimer's can provide patients with comfort, dignity, and independence for a longer period of time and can encourage and assist their caregivers as well.

It is important to understand that none of these medications stops the disease itself. Volunteers—people with Alzheimer's or mild cognitive impairment and healthy individuals—are needed to participate in Alzheimer's clinical research (see below).

Treatment for Mild to Moderate Alzheimer's

Medications called cholinesterase inhibitors are prescribed for mild to moderate Alzheimer's disease. These drugs may help delay or prevent symptoms from becoming worse for a limited time and may help control some behavioral symptoms. The medications include: Razadyne® (galantamine), Exelon® (rivastigmine), and Aricept® (donepezil). Another drug, Cognex® (tacrine), was the first approved cholinesterase inhibitor but is no longer available due to safety concerns.

Scientists do not yet fully understand how cholinesterase inhibitors work to treat Alzheimer's disease, but research indicates that they prevent the breakdown of acetylcholine, a brain chemical believed to be important for memory and thinking. As Alzheimer's progresses, the brain produces less and less acetylcholine; therefore, cholinesterase inhibitors may eventually lose their effect.

No published study directly compares these drugs. Because they work in a similar way, switching from one of these drugs to another probably will not produce significantly different results. However, an Alzheimer's patient may respond better to one drug than another.

Treatment for Moderate to Severe Alzheimer's

A medication known as Namenda® (memantine), an N-methyl D-aspartate (NMDA) antagonist, is prescribed to treat moderate to severe Alzheimer's disease. This drug's main effect is to delay progression of some of the symptoms of moderate to severe Alzheimer's. It may allow patients to maintain certain daily functions a little longer than they would without the medication. For example, Namenda® may help a patient in the later stages of the disease maintain his or her ability to use the bathroom independently for several more months, a benefit for both patients and caregivers.

Namenda® is believed to work by regulating glutamate, an important brain chemical. When produced in excessive amounts, glutamate may lead to brain cell death. Because NMDA antagonists work very differently from cholinesterase inhibitors, the two types of drugs can be prescribed in combination. The FDA has also approved Aricept® for the treatment of moderate to severe Alzheimer's disease.

Dosage and Side Effects

Doctors usually start patients at low drug doses and gradually increase the dosage based on how well a patient tolerates the drug. There is some evidence that certain patients may benefit from higher doses of the cholinesterase inhibitors. However, the higher the dose, the more likely are side effects.

Patients should be monitored when a drug is started. Report any unusual symptoms to the prescribing doctor right away. It is important to follow the doctor's instructions when taking any medication, including vitamins and herbal supplements. Also, let the doctor know before adding or changing any medications.

Behavioral Changes

As the disease progresses, a person with dementia may experience a variety of problems, like sleeplessness, agitation, wandering, anxiety, anger, and depression. Drug and non-drug treatments are available to manage these symptoms. Treating behavioral symptoms often makes people with Alzheimer's more comfortable and helps caregivers keep them safe.

Many people find the changes in behavior caused by Alzheimer's to be the most challenging and distressing effect of the disease. The chief cause of behavioral symptoms is the progressive deterioration of brain cells. However, medication, environmental influences, and some medical conditions also can cause symptoms or make them worse.

In early stages, people may experience behavior and personality changes such as:

- Irritability
- Anxiety
- Depression
- In later stages, other symptoms may occur including:
- Anger
- Agitation
- Aggression
- General emotional distress
- Physical or verbal outbursts
- Restlessness, pacing, shredding paper or tissues
- Hallucinations (seeing, hearing or feeling things that are not really there)
- Delusions (firmly held belief in things that are not true)
- Sleep disturbances

Triggering Situations

Events or changes in a person's surroundings often play a role in triggering behavioral symptoms. Change can be stressful for anyone and can be especially difficult for a person with Alzheimer's disease. It can increase the fear and fatigue of trying to make sense out of an increasingly confusing world.

Situations affecting behavior may include:

- Moving to a new residence or nursing home
- Changes in a familiar environment or caregiver arrangements
- Misperceived threats
- Admission to a hospital
- Being asked to bathe or change clothes
- Identifying what has triggered a behavior can often help in selecting the best approach to deal with it.

Medical Evaluation

Everyone who develops behavior changes should receive a thorough medical evaluation, especially if symptoms appear suddenly. Even though the chief cause of behavioral symptoms is the effect of Alzheimer's disease on the brain, an examination may reveal other treatable conditions that are contributing to the behavior.

Contributing conditions may include:

- Drug side effects. Many people with Alzheimer's take prescription medications for other health issues. Drug side effects or interactions among drugs can affect behavior.
- Discomfort from infections or other conditions. As the disease gets worse, those with Alzheimer's have increasing difficulty communicating with others about their experience. As a result, they may be unable to report symptoms of common illnesses. Pain from infections of the urinary tract, ear or sinuses may lead to restlessness or agitation. Discomfort from a full bladder, constipation, or feeling too hot or too cold also may be expressed through behavior.
- Uncorrected problems with hearing or vision. These can contribute to confusion and frustration and foster a sense of isolation.

Non-Drug Approaches

Non-drug approaches to managing behavior symptoms promote physical and emotional comfort. Many of these strategies aim to identify and address needs that the person with Alzheimer's may have difficulty expressing as the disease progresses. Non-drug approaches should always be tried first.

Steps to developing successful non-drug treatments include:

Recognizing that the person is not just "acting mean or ornery," but is having further symptoms of the disease

Identifying the cause and how the symptom may relate to the experience of the person with Alzheimer's

Changing the environment to resolve challenges and obstacles to comfort, security and ease of mind

Coping Tips

Monitor personal comfort. Check for pain, hunger, thirst, constipation, full bladder, fatigue, infections and skin irritation. Maintain a comfortable room temperature.

Avoid being confrontational or arguing about facts. For example, if a person expresses a wish to go visit a parent who died years ago, don't point out that the parent is dead. Instead, say, "Your mother is a wonderful person. I would like to see her too."

Redirect the person's attention. Try to remain flexible, patient and supportive by responding to the emotion, not the behavior.

Create a calm environment. Avoid noise, glare, insecure space and too much background distraction, including television.

Allow adequate rest between stimulating events.

Provide a security object.

Acknowledge requests, and respond to them.

Look for reasons behind each behavior. Consult a physician to identify any causes related to medications or illness.

Explore various solutions.

Don't take the behavior personally, and share your experiences with others.

Medications for BehavioralSsymptoms

If non-drug approaches fail after being applied consistently, introducing medications may be appropriate for individuals with severe symptoms or who have the potential to harm themselves or others. While prescription medications can be effective in some situations, they must be used carefully and are most effective when combined with non-drug approaches.

When considering use of medications, it is important to understand that no drugs are specifically approved by the U.S. Food and Drug Administration (FDA) to treat behavioral and psychiatric dementia symptoms. Some of the examples discussed below represent "off label" use, a medical practice in which a physician may prescribe a drug for a different purpose than the ones for which it is approved.

Medication examples

Some medications commonly used to treat behavioral and psychiatric symptoms of Alzheimer's disease, listed in alphabetical order by generic name, include the following:

- Antidepressants for low mood and irritability:
- citalopram (Celexa)
- fluoxetine (Prozac)
- paroxeine (Paxil)
- sertraline (Zoloft)

- trazodone (Desyrel)

Anxiolytics for anxiety, restlessness, verbally disruptive behavior and resistance:

- lorazepam (Ativan)
- oxazepam (Serax)

Antipsychotic medications for hallucinations, delusions, aggression, agitation, hostility and uncooperativeness:

- aripiprazole (Abilify)
- clozapine (Clozaril)
- haloperidol (Haldol)
- olanzapine (Zyprexa)
- quetiapine (Seroquel)
- risperidone (Risperdal)
- ziprasidone (Geodon)

Based on scientific evidence, as well as governmental warnings and guidance from care oversight bodies, individuals with dementia should use antipsychotic medications only under one of the following conditions:

- Behavioral symptoms are due to mania or psychosis
- The symptoms present a danger to the person or others
- The person is experiencing inconsolable or persistent distress, a significant decline in function or substantial difficulty receiving needed care

Antipsychotic medications should not be used to sedate or restrain persons with dementia. The minimum dosage should be used for the minimum amount of time possible. Adverse side effects require careful monitoring.

Although antipsychotics are the most frequently used medications for agitation, some physicians may prescribe a seizure medication/mood stabilizer, such as: carbamazepine (Tegretol).

Clinical Trials

Before any new medicine can be used to treat patients, it must be thoroughly tested to make sure it is safe and effective. Doctors who specialize in research conduct clinical trials to evaluate new medicines as well as other treatments, like exercise, diet, and even education programs to better treat—and hopefully one day prevent—Alzheimer's disease.

Thousands of people with Alzheimer's — as well as people who do not have the disease — are needed in clinical trials. Many study volunteers say this is one way they can directly be part of the fight against Alzheimer's.

Clinical trials are part of clinical research and at the heart of all medical advances. Clinical trials look at new ways to prevent, detect, or treat disease. Treatments might be new drugs or new combinations of drugs, new surgical procedures or devices, or new ways to use existing treatments. The goal of clinical trials is to determine if a new test or treatment works and is safe. Clinical trials can also look at other aspects of care, such as improving the quality of life for people with chronic illnesses.

People participate in clinical trials for a variety of reasons. Healthy volunteers say they participate to help others and to contribute to moving science forward. Participants with an illness or disease also participate to help others, but also to possibly receive the newest treatment and to have the additional care and attention from the clinical trial staff. Clinical trials offer hope for many people and an opportunity to help researchers find better treatments for others in the future.

Clinical Research

Clinical research is medical research that involves people like you. People volunteer to participate in carefully conducted investigations that ultimately uncover better ways to treat, prevent, diagnose, and understand human disease. Clinical research includes trials that test new treatments and therapies as well as long-term natural history studies, which provide valuable information about how disease and health progress.

The idea for a clinical research study — also known as a clinical trial — often originates in the laboratory. After researchers test new therapies or procedures in the laboratory and in animal studies, the most promising experimental treatments are moved into clinical trials, which are conducted in phases. During a trial, more information is gained about an experimental treatment, its risks, and its effectiveness.

Clinical research is conducted according to a plan known as a protocol. The protocol is carefully designed to safeguard the participants' health and answer specific research questions. A protocol describes the following:

- Who is eligible to participate in the trial
- Details about tests, procedures, medications, and dosages
- The length of the study and what information will be gathered

A clinical study is led by a principal investigator (PI), who is often a doctor. Members of the research team regularly monitor the participants' health to determine the study's safety and effectiveness.

Most, but not all, clinical trials in the United States are approved and monitored by an Institutional Review Board (IRB) in order to ensure that the risks are minimal and are worth any potential benefits. An IRB is an independent committee that consists of physicians, statisticians, and members of the community who ensure that clinical trials are ethical and that the rights of participants are protected. Potential research participants should ask the sponsor or research coordinator whether the research they are considering participating in was reviewed by an IRB.

Clinical trials are sponsored or funded by various organizations or individuals, including physicians, foundations, medical institutions, voluntary groups, and pharmaceutical companies, as well as federal agencies such as the National Institutes of Health and the Department of Veterans Affairs.

Informed Consent

Informed consent is the process of providing potential participants with the key facts about a clinical trial before they decide whether to participate. The process of informed consent (providing additional information) continues throughout the study. To help someone decide whether or not to participate, members of the research team explain the details of the study. Translation or interpretive assistance can be provided for participants with limited English proficiency. The research team provides an informed consent document that includes details about the study, such as its purpose, duration, required procedures, and who to contact for further information. The informed consent document also explains risks and potential benefits. The participant then decides whether to sign the document. Informed consent is not a contract. Volunteers are free to withdraw from the study completely or to refuse particular treatments or tests at any time. Sometimes, however, this will make them ineligible to continue the study.

Types of Clinical Trials

There are different types of clinical trials.
- Natural history studies provide valuable information about how disease and health progress
- Prevention trials look for better ways to prevent a disease in people who have never had the disease or to prevent the disease from

returning. Better approaches may include medicines, vaccines, or lifestyle changes, among other things.

- Screening trials test the best way to detect certain diseases or health conditions.
- Diagnostic trials determine better tests or procedures for diagnosing a particular disease or condition.
- Treatment trials test new treatments, new combinations of drugs, or new approaches to surgery or radiation therapy.
- Quality of life trials (or supportive care trials) explore and measure ways to improve the comfort and quality of life of people with a chronic illness.

Clinical trials are conducted in "phases." Each phase has a different purpose and helps researchers answer different questions.

- Phase I trials: Researchers test an experimental drug or treatment in a small group of people (20–80) for the first time. The purpose is to evaluate its safety and identify side effects.
- Phase II trials: The experimental drug or treatment is administered to a larger group of people (100–300) to determine its effectiveness and to further evaluate its safety.
- Phase III trials: The experimental drug or treatment is administered to large groups of people (1,000–3,000) to confirm its effectiveness, monitor side effects, compare it with standard or equivalent treatments, and collect information that will allow the experimental drug or treatment to be used safely.
- Phase IV trials: After a drug is approved by the FDA and made available to the public, researchers track its safety, seeking more information about a drug or treatment's risks, benefits, and optimal use.

Typically, clinical trials compare a new product or therapy with another that already exists to determine if the new one is as successful as, or better than, the existing one. In some studies, participants may be assigned to receive a placebo (an inactive product that resembles the test product, but without its treatment value).

Comparing a new product with a placebo can be the fastest and most reliable way to demonstrate the new product's therapeutic effectiveness. However, placebos are not used if a patient would be put at risk — particularly in the study of treatments for serious illnesses — by not having effective therapy. Most of these studies compare new products with an approved therapy. Potential participants are told if placebos will be used in the study before they enter a trial.

Randomization is the process by which two or more alternative treatments are assigned to volunteers by chance rather than by choice. This is done to avoid any bias with investigators assigning volunteers to one group or another.   The results of each treatment are compared at specific points during a trial, which may last for years. When one treatment is found superior, the trial is stopped so that the fewest volunteers receive the less beneficial treatment.

In single-or double-blind studies, also called single- or double-masked studies, the participants do not know which medicine is being used, so they can describe what happens without bias. "Blind" (or "masked") studies are designed to prevent members of the research team or study participants from influencing the results. This allows scientifically accurate conclusions. In single-blind ("single-masked") studies, only the patient is not told what is being administered. In a double-blind study, only the pharmacist knows; members of the research team are not told which patients are getting which medication, so that their observations will not be biased. If medically necessary, however, it is always possible to find out what the patient is taking.

Many different types of people participate in clinical trials. Some are healthy, while others may have illnesses. A healthy volunteer is a person with no known significant health problems who participates in clinical research to test a new drug, device, or intervention. Research procedures with healthy volunteers are designed to develop new knowledge, not to provide direct benefit to study participants. Healthy volunteers have always played an important role in research.

Healthy volunteers are needed for several reasons. When developing a new technique, such as a blood test or imaging device, healthy volunteers (formerly called "normal volunteers") help define the limits of "normal." These volunteers serve as controls for patient groups and are often matched to patients on characteristics such as age, gender, or family relationship. They receive the same test, procedure, or drug the patient group receives. Investigators learn about the disease process by comparing the patient group to the healthy volunteers.

Factors like how much of your time is needed, discomfort you may feel, or risk involved depends on the trial. While some require minimal amounts of time and effort, other studies may require a major commitment in time and effort on behalf of the volunteer, and may involve some discomfort. The research procedure may also carry some risk. The consent process for healthy volunteers includes a detailed discussion of the study's procedures and tests.

A patient volunteer has a known health problem and participates in research to better understand, diagnose, treat, or cure that disease or condition. Research procedures with a patient volunteer help develop new knowledge. These procedures may or may not benefit the study participants.

Patient volunteers may be involved in studies similar to those in which healthy volunteers participate. These studies involve drugs, devices, or interventions designed to prevent, treat, or cure disease. Although these studies may provide direct benefit to patient volunteers, the main aim is to prove, by scientific means, the effects and limitations of the experimental treatment. Consequently, some patients serve as controls by not taking the test drug, or by receiving test doses of the drug large enough only to show that it is present, but not at a level that can treat the condition. A study's benefits may be indirect for the volunteers but may help others.

All clinical trials have guidelines about who can participate, called Inclusion/Exclusion Criteria. Factors that allow someone to participate in a clinical trial are "inclusion criteria." Those that exclude or not allow participation are "exclusion criteria." These criteria are based on factors such as age, gender, the type and stage of a disease, previous treatment history, and other medical conditions. Before joining a clinical trial, a participant must qualify for the study. Some research studies seek participants with illnesses or conditions to be studied in the clinical trial, while others need healthy volunteers.

Some studies need both types. Inclusion and exclusion criteria are not used to reject people personally; rather, the criteria are used to identify appropriate participants and keep them safe, and to help ensure that researchers can find new information they need.

Risks and Benefits

Clinical trials involve risks, just as routine medical care and the activities of daily living. When weighing the risks of research, you can consider two important factors:

- the degree of harm that could result from participating in the study, and
- the chance of any harm occurring.

Most clinical studies pose the risk of minor discomfort, which lasts only a short time. However, some study participants experience complications that require medical attention. In rare cases, participants have been seriously injured or have died of complications resulting from their participation in trials of experimental therapies. The specific risks associated with a research protocol are described in detail in the informed consent document, which participants are asked to sign before participating in research. Also, a member of the research team explains the major risks of participating in a study and will answer any questions you have about the study. Before deciding to participate, carefully consider possible risks and benefits.

Well-designed and well-executed clinical trials provide the best approach for participants to:

- Play an active role in their health care.
- Gain access to new research treatments before they are widely available.
- Receive regular and careful medical attention from a research team that includes doctors and other health professionals.
- Help others by contributing to medical research.

Risks to participating in clinical trials include the following:

- There may be unpleasant, serious, or even life-threatening side effects to experimental treatment.
- The study may require more time and attention than standard treatment would, including visits to the study site, more blood tests, more treatments, hospital stays, or complex dosage requirements.

Ethical Guidelines

The goal of clinical research is to develop knowledge that improves human health or increases understanding of human biology. People who participate in clinical research make it possible for this to occur. The path to finding out if a new drug is safe or effective is to test it on patient volunteers. By placing some people at risk of harm for the good of others, clinical research has the potential to exploit patient volunteers. The purpose of ethical guidelines is both to protect patient volunteers and to preserve the integrity of the science. Ethical guidelines in place today were primarily a response to past research abuses. If the participant decides to enroll in the trial, the informed consent document will be signed. Informed consent is not a contract. Volunteers are free to withdraw from the study at any time.

IRB Review

Most, but not all, clinical trials in the United States are approved and monitored by an Institutional Review Board (IRB) in order to ensure that the risks are minimal and are worth any potential benefits. An IRB is an independent committee that consists of physicians, statisticians, and members of the community who ensure that clinical trials are ethical and that the rights of participants are protected. Potential research participants should ask the sponsor or research coordinator whether the research they are considering participating in was reviewed by an IRB.

IMPACT ON CAREGIVERS

Because of caregiving duties, women are likely to experience adverse consequences in the workplace. Nearly 19 percent of women Alzheimer's caregivers had to quit work either to become a caregiver or because their caregiving duties became too burdensome.

In 2013, 15.5 million family and friends provided 17.7 billion hours of unpaid care to those with Alzheimer's and other dementias – care valued at $220.2 billion, which is nearly eight times the total revenue of McDonald's in 2012. More than 60 percent of Alzheimer's and dementia caregivers are women.

All caregivers of people with Alzheimer's – both women and men – face a devastating toll. Due to the physical and emotional burden of caregiving, Alzheimer's and dementia caregivers had $9.3 billion in additional health care costs of their own in 2013. Nearly 60 percent of Alzheimer's and dementia caregivers rate the emotional stress of caregiving as high or very high, and more than one-third report symptoms of depression.

10

Chronic and Disabling Disease

In 1996, Claude Lenfant, M.D., director of the National Heart, Lung and Blood Institute at the time, presented the following testimony to the Senate Committee on Labor and Human Resources*:

Chronic and disabling diseases affect millions of Americans in all strata of society. They constitute an incalculable public health burden in terms of pain and suffering, loss of function, and healthcare resource utilization. Some (e.g., cystic fibrosis, cerebral palsy) are present at birth; others (e.g., Crohn's disease, sarcoidosis) become manifest in youth or middle age; others (e.g., osteoporosis, macular degeneration) strike in old age; and still others, like alcoholism, appear through all phases of life. Many ultimately lead to death; all compromise the patient's quality of life. The demographics of our population are changing rapidly, and it is clear that with increasing life expectancy come increasing opportunities for people to fall prey to chronic and disabling diseases. This is the "epidemic" of the modern age

The biological, behavioral, and societal consequences of these diseases are manifold, and so are their causes. Both genes and environment contribute to every pathological process, but each chronic disease is unique in terms of how it is likely to come about and who may be affected. Down syndrome, for instance, is almost entirely genetically determined. At the other end of the spectrum, cirrhosis and chronic obstructive pulmonary disease are strongly influenced by environmental exposures to alcohol and tobacco. In between are widespread disorders, such as hypertension, that confound us because they stem from complex and interactive factors.

---

* http://www.hhs.gov/asl/testify/t960307c.html

247

Among the most daunting challenges that we face are the increasingly prevalent chronic diseases that reflect, to a great extent, the fruit of our efforts to combat more short-lived maladies. In the case of diabetes, for instance, the discovery of insulin mitigated what had been a certain death sentence for its victims. However, the long-term survival of diabetic patients has given rise to a very large population of Americans who not only require chronic treatment, but also are subject to an array of devastating complications, such as heart attack, stroke, kidney failure, limb amputation, and blindness. Similarly, our remarkable success at saving babies born before their time has left us with a host of problems, including the chronic lung disease bronchopulmonary dysplasia, that must be addressed. What we have learned has benefited society enormously, but we still have far to go.

We have the tools to solve these problems. Modem approaches to scientific investigation are now revolutionizing our ability to understand how the human body functions at the most fundamental level of the cell and the molecule. By capitalizing on these new opportunities and integrating their findings into the vast body of knowledge acquired over the past century, we can substantially decrease the burden of disease.

Because chronic and disabling diseases affect every part of the human body and every age group, they are the concern of all the NIH Institutes and Centers. A coordinated research effort in this area ensures that multiple perspectives are brought to bear on these diseases, and that knowledge gained in one organ system stimulates new approaches to the study of other systems.

SICKLE CELL DISEASE

Sickle cell disease is one of the most tenacious and inexorable of chronic diseases in that afflicts its victims from cradle to grave. It is characterized by recurrent bouts of pain ("crises"), chronic anemia related to accelerated destruction of red blood cells, increased susceptibility to certain infections, and acute or chronic damage to various organs. Children inherit sickle cell disease when the gene for defective ("sickle") hemoglobin is passed on from both parents. In this country the illness occurs predominantly, but not exclusively, in persons of African ancestry; about 50,000 to 60,000 American blacks are affected. Health-care costs for patients with sickle cell disease can be extremely high, quality of life is impaired, and loss of time from school or employment is common. Thus, sickle cell disease is a problem of significant medical, psychological, social, and economic importance.

Although research on sickle cell disease began less than 25 years ago, progress has been rapid. Few patients used to survive beyond the third decade, but now many are living into their 50s and beyond. In 1977 sickle cell disease became the first human malady to be described at the level of DNA and RNA. Breakthroughs that rapidly followed made it possible to apply gene mapping techniques to prenatal diagnosis and to use placental tissue rather than fetal blood samples for this purpose. This substantially increased the safety of prenatal diagnosis for sickle cell disease, and rapidly led to the application of molecular genetics for prenatal diagnosis of other inherited diseases.

At the same time, basic research supported in scientific laboratories throughout the country brought a tremendous revolution in our understanding of sickle cell disease at the molecular level.

One of the earliest NIH programs focused on research to determine the mechanisms that regulate the "switch" from fetal to adult hemoglobin during infancy. It had been recognized for some time that sickle cell patients who were fortunate enough to have inherited a tendency to continue producing fetal hemoglobin beyond the first year of fife had relatively benign disease. Therefore, it seemed logical to pursue therapeutic modalities that would enable patients producing adult sickle hemoglobin to "switch back" to producing normal fetal hemoglobin. This research catalyzed the field of molecular biology, and became the cornerstone for development of new therapeutic approaches. It produced news headlines last year when the results of a landmark clinical trial showed that administration of hydroxyurea, a common chemotherapeutic agent that boosts fetal hemoglobin production, not only reduces the frequency of crises and their attendant hospitalizations, but also reduces episodes of acute chest syndrome, a pneumonia-like complication, and the need for blood transfusions.

Very early on, it became apparent that although much was known about the molecular basis of sickle cell disease, little was known about its natural history or clinical course. Only the sickest patients were described in the medical literature, and most clinical reports of patient outcomes were anecdotal and retrospective. The Cooperative Study of Sickle Cell Disease addressed many of these unknowns. It clarified issues of growth and maturation patterns among children with sickle cell disease; defined the causes of death in the pediatric population; described the epidemiology of painful episodes and documented, for the first time, that the frequency with which such crises occur is a predictor of premature death in adult patients; and pointed out the risks of alloimmunization for sickle cell patients receiving repeated blood transfusions. This research program redoubled efforts to search for new therapeutic agents, and also provided a model from Comprehensive Sickle Cell Centers, for a revised management approach that places the central focus on the patient. Care that was previously fragmented, impersonal, and episodic has been replaced with a team approach, involving a cadre of trained personnel that includes not only physicians, but also nurses, social workers, psychologists, nutritionists, counselors, and allied health professionals.

Subsequent clinical research demonstrated the value of prophylactic penicillin in preventing major infections in infants and young children. Before that discovery, approximately 30 percent of sickle cell deaths occurred before 5 years of age, most in children under the age of 2, and the majority were due to pneumococcal infection. This work also provided impetus for recommending that d newborns be screened for sickle cell disease, which is currently being carried out in 42 states. Infants at risk could then be referred for comprehensive care, and prophylactic penicillin therapy could be given by 3 months of age. A follow up study determined that this therapy can safely be discontinued in most patients at 5 years of age, thereby decreasing the risk of promoting drug-resistant infections in this vulnerable population.

"We see a new era of optimism for treating and, indeed, curing sickle cell disease patients, because we are on the threshold of moving molecular medicine even closer to the bedside. Gene therapy and bone marrow transplantation offer great hopes for eliminating this disease. Bone marrow transplantation has been successfully used by several investigators in Europe, as well as a small number in the United States. Although early reports are Promising, patient selection, donor availability, and complications of the procedure continue to be potential problems that prevent widespread use of this therapeutic modality today"

Basic research on gene therapy is advancing, with the possibility of inserting normal genes for hemoglobin production into bone marrow precursor or stem cells, thus enabling the production of normal hemoglobin. Our ability to obtain highly enriched quantities of stem cells from cord blood, peripheral blood, and bone mar-row will facilitate continued advances in gene transfer strategies. However, the efficiency of gene transfer must be improved before this procedure has the potential for therapeutic benefit in sickle cell disease. This approach is receiving active attention by many researchers around the country, who are optimistic that a cure for sickle cell disease can be achieved within the next decade.

ARTHRITIC DISORDERS

Arthritic disorders are chronic and disabling diseases that occur at all ages, destroy the quality of life, and require long-term medical care. By the year 2020, when the baby boomer generation approaches the prime year of onset of certain forms of arthritis (osteoarthritis), a large percentage of the population could be afflicted. Studies are focusing on many of the over one hundred forms of arthritis-related diseases, with major emphasis on rheumatoid arthritis, systemic lupus erythematosus, and osteoarthritis.

Rheumatoid arthritis is a chronic inflammatory disease that usually occurs in early adulthood or middle age. The joints of the body become painful, swollen, stiff, and in severe cases, deformed. Rheumatoid arthritis involves the hands, wrists, elbows, shoulders, and knees. The disease can also cause widespread inflammation in blood vessels throughout the body.

Scientists have discovered that white blood cells have specific cell adhesion molecules that facilitate their movement into joints. Considerable evidence has also indicated that chemicals, such as tumor necrosis factor-alpha and interleukin- 1, are released by white blood cells that invade the joints and cause the inflammation. This is thought to indicate that rheumatoid arthritis is a form of a self-destructive, or autoimmune, process. Efforts are being directed at blocking the movement of white blood cells into joints, as well as blocking the action of the chemicals released by the white blood cells, thus preventing or controlling inflammation.

Other research efforts are focusing on the growth of new blood vessels (angiogenesis), which can deliver white blood cells that cause the destruction of joints. A novel angiogenesis inhibitor that can slow and even prevent the chronic inflammation of arthritis in several experimental disease models has recently been identified. The inhibitor is currently undergoing preliminary clinical trials. Better understanding of the angiogenesis process, its role in destructive diseases such as rheumatoid arthritis, and the effects of angiogenesis inhibition could provide new and possibly more effective means to manage a wide range of joint problems.

Another arthritic disorder, systemic lupus erythematosus, also called SLE or lupus, is a disorder of the immune system in which the body produces abnormal antibodies(autoantibodies) that react against the person's own tissues. Lupus can affect many parts of the body including the skin, joints, heart, lungs, kidneys, and nervous system. Lupus primarily affects women of childbearing age, at a ratio of nine women to one man, and it is three times more common in black women than in write women.

Over the past several years scientists have developed more sensitive laboratory tests for autoantibodies in blood serum, enabling recognition of milder forms of lupus. Hormone-like chemicals called cytokines, which are produced by white blood cells, marshal the body's immune response to foreign substances and stimulate the production of multiple autoantibodies. Researchers hope to learn more about environmental and other factors that result in the production of harmful antibodies so that they can develop intervention strategies.

Research into the genetic basis of lupus is also ongoing. In a recently identified mutant mouse strain that develops a lupus-like illness, there is a defect in one of the genes that causes apoptosis, a normal process by which the body eliminates unnecessary, damaged, or potentially harmful cells. When this defective gene is replaced with a normal gene, the mice no longer develop signs of lupus. Better understanding of the role of apoptosis in lupus may lead to new, targeted treatments for humans. Other researchers have found various features of lupus are affected by distinct but additive, genetic contributions. This work is important because a similar effort to identify genetic susceptibility is now being made in humans.

Long-term clinical trials by NIH intramural scientists using various immunosuppressive drugs to treat lupus nephritis—a form of lupus that can be life-threatening-have demonstrated that prednisone combined with intravenous cyclophosphamide is very beneficial. This approach has now become standard clinical practice for the treatment of patients. These scientists are now exploring other drugs as well as biological agents, such as new monoclonal antibodies, for treating lupus nephritis. Such agents would enable physicians to circumvent the toxic side-effects associated with powerful immunosuppressive drugs. At the present time, women with lupus are generally advised not to take any medications that contain estrogen in the belief that it will worsen their disease.

It remains a puzzle as to why in patients such as those with rheumatoid arthritis and systemic lupus erythematosus, the body's own immune system reacts against other cells and tissues. The major histocompatibility complex (a group of inherited genes) has emerged as the single most predisposing factor for autoimmune diseases ranging from rheumatoid arthritis and lupus to insulin dependent diabetes mellitus. Yet, in spite of this striking association and the abundant information about the structure of major histocompatibility complex molecules, mechanisms underlying their role in determining whether or not the body's own cells will be tolerated or attacked, as in the above-mentioned autoimmune diseases, remain a mystery. The major histocompatibility complex may affect disease predisposition through several mechanisms. The increased capacity to predict the interaction between the major histocompatibility complex and small components of proteins called peptides, and the availability of methods to test for major histocompatibility complex involvement have provided new and challenging opportunities for identification and analysis of self and foreign peptides in the production of autoimmunity.

Osteoarthritis, or degenerative joint disease, is the most common form of arthritis and occurs mainly in older persons. Osteoarthritis affects cartilage, the protective material that covers the ends of bones, causing it to fray, wear, and, in extreme cases, disappear entirely, leaving a bone-on-bone joint.

It's characterized by joint problems related to bone-on-bone contact of the joints that is usually caused when a joint loses the cushioning effects of either its protective tissue or fluids. Osteoarthritis can also by caused by wear and tear from repeated pressure or too much weight. This condition can be highly painful and can limit the range of motion in the affected joints.

Your risk for experiencing osteoarthritis increases with your age. It also increases with weight you carry, whether that's your body weight or extra weight of carrying heavy things for your job or recreation (for example, regularly hiking with a heavy backpack). That is why it's important to take caution when repeatedly carrying heavy items and maintain your weight below 25 on the body mass index (BMI). You can use the BMI calculator at the bottom of the page to determine your BMI. The goal is to reduce the pressure and wear and tear on the cartilage and other cushioning tissues in the joint.

Osteoarthritis can cause pain stiffness, and swelling of the joints and loss of function. Disability results most often from disease in the knees, hips, and spine. About one-third of adults in the United States have x-ray evidence of osteoarthritis in the hand, foot, knee, or hip-, and by age 65, as much as 75 percent of the population has x-ray evidence of osteoarthritis in at least one of these sites. Research into the causes and treatment of osteoarthritis is multi-faceted and includes population-based studies, basic research at the molecular and cellular level, and investigations into designing more effective and longer lasting artificial joint replacements.

Much of the basic research on osteoarthritis has focused on differences between the cells of normal and osteoarthritic cartilage. A key component of cartilage is collagen, a widely distributed connective and supportive tissue protein. This fiber-like protein has the ability to trap water and become sponge-like. The resiliency that collagen imparts to normal cartilage makes it possible for joints to withstand the pressure of body weight. The degradation of cartilage that leads to joint damage in osteoarthritis is sometimes caused by enzymes acting on collagen. As this enzymatic breakdown of collagen takes place, cartilage can become damaged by weight and other mechanical forces. Scientists have recently discovered inhibitors of these destructive enzymes. Several are being tested in small clinical trials supported by pharmaceutical firms in the United States and abroad. Other investigators are carrying out laboratory studies on molecular mechanisms to suppress collagenase genetically. Major efforts are also being expended in trying to understand how growth factors and bone and matrix morphogenic proteins, which are known to enhance cartilage formation, can be used therapeutically in osteoarthritis.

The current widespread use of joint replacements represents a singularly significant advance in the treatment of osteoarthritis. At present more than 120,000 artificial joints for hips are being implanted in the United States annually, the majority in patients with osteoarthritis. Past research has contributed to development of improved prostheses and joint replacement procedures. Current studies are attempting to identify causes of prosthesis failure and why various prostheses and particles released from prostheses cause bone resorption.

Many factors determine the pain, function, and quality of life of those with arthritis. Greater physical activity can reduce pain and improve function. However, physical activity remains an underused intervention, even though there are a variety of programs to help people with arthritis increase physical activity safely and with little pain. Self-management education can achieve similar positive outcomes by teaching people skills and techniques to deal with the day-to-day issues that result from arthritis. Weight loss among those who are overweight or obese also helps reduce symptoms of arthritis.

Prevention

Be physically active – Taking part in regular physical activity that keeps the body and joints in good working order. The U.S. Department of Health and Human Services (HHS) recommends that adults get at least two-and-a-half hours of moderate to vigorous physical activity each week. You don't have to do it all at once; you can spread this activity out over easy

30-minute increments, five days a week. Or you can choose from many activities and do them in bouts of 10 minutes. The HHS also advises doing muscle-strengthening exercises two or more days a week. Regular physical activity can also help you maintain a healthy weight.

If you've already been diagnosed with some type of arthritis, work with your health care provider on your treatment plan. Also, ask your health care provider about what level of regular physical activity is best for you.

Maintaining a healthy weight – To find out where you stand, use the BMI calculator on the bottom of this page. If your BMI is lower than 25, you can maintain your weight by eating healthy foods and getting regular physical activity. If you are overweight (your BMI is 25 or higher), combining a low-calorie, well-balanced diet with regular physical activity can help you let go of the extra weight. Always remember that healthy weight loss isn't just about a "diet" or "program." The key to success is ongoing lifestyle choices that include long-term changes in both daily eating and physical activity habits. Realistic goals with small and consistent wins will bring you back to a weight that is healthy for you.

Make a good team – Work closely with your health care provider, letting him or her know of any symptoms you're experiencing that could be related to arthritis or an autoimmune condition. Often, catching the disease early can make a big difference in your ability to control the symptoms.

CHRONIC BACK CONDITIONS

If you have lower back pain, you are not alone. About 80 percent of adults experience low back pain at some point in their lifetimes. It is the most common cause of job-related disability and a leading contributor to missed work days. In a large survey, more than a quarter of adults reported experiencing low back pain during the past 3 months.

Men and women are equally affected by low back pain, which can range in intensity from a dull, constant ache to a sudden, sharp sensation that leaves the person incapacitated. Pain can begin abruptly as a result of an accident or by lifting something heavy, or it can develop over time due to age-related changes of the spine. Sedentary lifestyles also can set the stage for low back pain, especially when a weekday routine of getting too little exercise is punctuated by strenuous weekend workout.

Most low back pain is acute, or short term, and lasts a few days to a few weeks. It tends to resolve on its own with self-care and there is no residual loss of function. The majority of acute low back pain is mechanical in nature, meaning that there is a disruption in the way the components of the back (the spine, muscle, intervertebral discs, and nerves) fit together and move.

Subacute low back pain is defined as pain that lasts between 4 and 12 weeks.

Chronic back pain is defined as pain that persists for 12 weeks or longer, even after an initial injury or underlying cause of acute low back pain has been treated. About 20 percent of people affected by acute low back pain develop chronic low back pain with persistent symptoms at one year. In some cases, treatment successfully relieves chronic low back pain, but in other cases pain persists despite medical and surgical treatment.

The magnitude of the burden from low back pain has grown worse in recent years. In 1990, a study ranking the most burdensome conditions in the U.S. in terms of mortality or poor health as a result of disease put low back pain in sixth place; in 2010, low back pain jumped to third place, with only ischemic heart disease and chronic obstructive pulmonary disease ranking higher.

The lower back where most back pain occurs includes the five vertebrae (referred to as L_1-L_5) in the lumbar region, which supports much of the weight of the upper body. The spaces between the vertebrae are maintained by round, rubbery pads called intervertebral discs that act like shock absorbers throughout the spinal column to cushion the bones as the body moves. Bands of tissue known as ligaments hold the vertebrae in place, and tendons attach the muscles to the spinal column. Thirty-one pairs of nerves are rooted to the spinal cord and they control body movements and transmit signals from the body to the brain.

Causes

The vast majority of low back pain is mechanical in nature. In many cases, low back pain is associated with spondylosis, a term that refers to the general degeneration of the spine associated with normal wear and tear that occurs in the joints, discs, and bones of the spine as people get older. Some examples of mechanical causes of low back pain include:

Sprains and strains account for most acute back pain. Sprains are caused by overstretching or tearing ligaments, and strains are tears in tendon or muscle. Both can occur from twisting or lifting something improperly, lifting something too heavy, or overstretching. Such movements may also trigger spasms in back muscles, which can also be painful.

Intervertebral disc degeneration is one of the most common mechanical causes of low back pain, and it occurs when the usually rubbery discs lose integrity as a normal process of aging. In a healthy back, intervertebral discs provide height and allow bending, flexion, and torsion of the lower back. As the discs deteriorate, they lose their cushioning ability.

Herniated or ruptured discs can occur when the intervertebral discs become compressed and bulge outward (herniation) or rupture, causing low back pain.

Radiculopathy is a condition caused by compression, inflammation and/or injury to a spinal nerve root. Pressure on the nerve root results in pain, numbness, or a tingling sensation that travels or radiates to other areas of the body that are served by that nerve. Radiculopathy may occur when spinal stenosis or a herniated or ruptured disc compresses the nerve root.

Sciatica is a form of radiculopathy caused by compression of the sciatic nerve, the large nerve that travels through the buttocks and extends down the back of the leg. This compression causes shock-like or burning low back pain combined with pain through the buttocks and down one leg, occasionally reaching the foot. In the most extreme cases, when the nerve is pinched between the disc and the adjacent bone, the symptoms may involve not only pain, but numbness and muscle weakness in the leg because of interrupted nerve signaling. The condition may also be caused by a tumor or cyst that presses on the sciatic nerve or its roots.

Spondylolisthesis is a condition in which a vertebra of the lower spine slips out of place, pinching the nerves exiting the spinal column.

A traumatic injury, such as from playing sports, car accidents, or a fall can injure tendons, ligaments or muscle resulting in low back pain. Traumatic injury may also cause the spine to become overly compressed, which in turn can cause an intervertebral disc to rupture or herniate, exerting pressure on any of the nerves rooted to the spinal cord. When spinal nerves become compressed and irritated, back pain and sciatica may result.

Spinal stenosis is a narrowing of the spinal column that puts pressure on the spinal cord and nerves that can cause pain or numbness with walking and over time leads to leg weakness and sensory loss.

Skeletal irregularities include scoliosis, a curvature of the spine that does not usually cause pain until middle age; lordosis, an abnormally accentuated arch in the lower back; and other congenital anomalies of the spine.

Low back pain is rarely related to serious underlying conditions, but when these conditions do occur, they require immediate medical attention. Serious underlying conditions include:

Infections are not a common cause of back pain. However, infections can cause pain when they involve the vertebrae, a condition called osteomyelitis; the intervertebral discs, called discitis; or the sacroiliac joints connecting the lower spine to the pelvis, called sacroiliitis.

Tumors are a relatively rare cause of back pain. Occasionally, tumors begin in the back, but more often they appear in the back as a result of cancer that has spread from elsewhere in the body.

Cauda equina syndrome is a serious but rare complication of a ruptured disc. It occurs when disc material is pushed into the spinal canal and compresses the bundle of lumbar and sacral nerve roots, causing loss of bladder and bowel control. Permanent neurological damage may result if this syndrome is left untreated.

Abdominal aortic aneurysms occur when the large blood vessel that supplies blood to the abdomen, pelvis, and legs becomes abnormally enlarged. Back pain can be a sign that the aneurysm is becoming larger and that the risk of rupture should be assessed.

Kidney stones can cause sharp pain in the lower back, usually on one side.

Other underlying conditions that predispose people to low back pain include:

Inflammatory diseases of the joints such as arthritis, including osteoarthritis and rheumatoid arthritis as well as spondylitis, an inflammation of the vertebrae, can also cause low back pain. Spondylitis is also called spondyloarthritis or spondyloarthropathy.

Osteoporosis is a metabolic bone disease marked by a progressive decrease in bone density and strength, which can lead to painful fractures of the vertebrae.

Endometriosis is the buildup of uterine tissue in places outside the uterus.

Fibromyalgia, a chronic pain syndrome involving widespread muscle pain and fatigue.

Risks

Beyond underlying diseases, certain other risk factors may elevate one's risk for low back pain, including:

Age: The first attack of low back pain typically occurs between the ages of 30 and 50, and back pain becomes more common with advancing age. As people grow older, loss of bone strength from osteoporosis can lead to fractures, and at the same time, muscle elasticity and tone decrease. The intervertebral discs begin to lose fluid and flexibility with age, which decreases their ability to cushion the vertebrae. The risk of spinal stenosis also increases with age.

Fitness level: Back pain is more common among people who are not physically fit. Weak back and abdominal muscles may not properly support the spine. "Weekend warriors"—people who go out and exercise a lot after being inactive all week—are more likely to suffer painful back injuries than people who make moderate physical activity a daily habit. Studies show that low-impact aerobic exercise is beneficial for the maintaining the integrity of intervertebral discs.

Pregnancy is commonly accompanied by low back pain, which results from pelvic changes and alterations in weight loading. Back symptoms almost always resolve postpartum.

Weight gain: Being overweight, obese, or quickly gaining significant amounts of weight can put stress on the back and lead to low back pain.

Genetics: Some causes of back pain, such as ankylosing spondylitis, a form of arthritis that involves fusion of the spinal joints leading to some immobility of the spine, have a genetic component.

Occupational risk factors: Having a job that requires heavy lifting, pushing, or pulling, particularly when it involves twisting or vibrating the spine, can lead to injury and back pain. An inactive job or a desk job may also lead to or contribute to pain, especially if you have poor posture or sit all day in a chair with inadequate back support.

Mental health factors: Pre-existing mental health issues such as anxiety and depression can influence how closely one focuses on their pain as well as their perception of its severity. Pain that becomes chronic also can contribute to the development of such psychological factors. Stress can affect the body in numerous ways, including causing muscle tension.

Backpack overload in children: Low back pain unrelated to injury or other known cause is unusual in pre-teen children. However, a backpack overloaded with schoolbooks and supplies can strain the back and cause muscle fatigue. The American Academy of Orthopaedic Surgeons recommends that a child's backpack should weigh no more than 15 to 20 percent of the child's body weight.

Diagnosis

A complete medical history and physical exam can usually identify any serious conditions that may be causing the pain. During the exam, a health care provider will ask about the onset, site, and severity of the pain; duration of symptoms and any limitations in movement; and history of previous episodes or any health conditions that might be related to the pain. Along with a thorough back examination, neurologic tests are conducted to determine the cause of pain and appropriate treatment. The cause of chronic lower back pain is often difficult to determine even after a thorough examination.

Imaging tests are not warranted in most cases. Under certain circumstances, however, imaging may be ordered to rule out specific causes of pain, including tumors and spinal stenosis. Imaging and other types of tests include:

X-ray is often the first imaging technique used to look for broken bones or an injured vertebra. X-rays show the bony structures and any vertebral misalignment or fractures. Soft tissues such as muscles, ligaments, or bulging discs are not visible on conventional x-rays.

Computerized tomography (CT) is used to see spinal structures that cannot be seen on conventional x-rays, such as disc rupture, spinal stenosis, or tumors. Using a computer, the CT scan creates a three-dimensional image from a series of two dimensional pictures.

Myelograms enhance the diagnostic imaging of x-rays and CT scans. In this procedure, a contrast dye is injected into the spinal canal, allowing spinal cord and nerve compression caused by herniated discs or fractures to be seen on an x-ray or CT scans.

Discography may be used when other diagnostic procedures fail to identify the cause of pain. This procedure involves the injection of a contrast dye into a spinal disc thought to be causing low back pain. The fluid's pressure in the disc will reproduce the person's symptoms if the disc is the cause. The dye helps to show the damaged areas on CT scans taken following the injection. Discography may provide useful information in cases where people are considering lumbar surgery or when their pain has not responded to conventional treatments.

Magnetic resonance imaging (MRI) uses a magnetic force instead of radiation to create a computer-generated image. Unlike x-ray, which shows only bony structures, MRI scans also produce images of soft tissues such as muscles, ligaments, tendons, and blood vessels. An MRI may be ordered if a problem such as infection, tumor, inflammation, disc herniation or rupture, or pressure on a nerve is suspected. MRI is a noninvasive way to identify a condition requiring prompt surgical treatment. However, in most instances, unless there are "red flags" in the history or physical exam, an MRI scan is not necessary during the early phases of low back pain.

Electrodiagnostics are procedures that, in the setting of low back pain, are primarily used to confirm whether a person has lumbar radiculopathy. The procedures include electromyography (EMG), nerve conduction studies (NCS), and evoked potential (EP) studies. EMG assesses the electrical activity in a muscle and can detect if muscle weakness results from a problem with the nerves that control the muscles. Very fine needles are inserted in muscles to measure electrical activity transmitted from the brain or spinal cord to a particular area of the body. NCSs are often performed along with EMG to exclude conditions that can mimic radiculopathy. In NCSs, two sets of electrodes are placed on the skin over the muscles. The first set provides a mild shock to stimulate the nerve that runs to a particular muscle. The second set records the nerve's electrical signals, and from this information nerve damage that slows conduction of the nerve signal can be detected. EP tests also involve two sets of electrodes—one set to stimulate a sensory nerve, and the other placed on the scalp to record the speed of nerve signal transmissions to the brain.

Bone scans are used to detect and monitor infection, fracture, or disorders in the bone. A small amount of radioactive material is injected into the bloodstream and will collect in the bones, particularly in areas with some abnormality. Scanner-generated images can be used to identify specific areas of irregular bone metabolism or abnormal blood flow, as well as to measure levels of joint disease.

Ultrasound imaging, also called ultrasound scanning or sonography, uses high-frequency sound waves to obtain images inside the body. The sound wave echoes are recorded and displayed as a real-time visual image. Ultrasound imaging can show tears in ligaments, muscles, tendons, and other soft tissue masses in the back.

Blood tests are not routinely used to diagnose the cause of back pain; however in some cases they may be ordered to look for indications of inflammation, infection, and/or the presence of arthritis. Potential tests include complete blood count, erythrocyte sedimentation rate, and C-reactive protein. Blood tests may also detect HLA-B27, a genetic marker in the blood that is more common in people with ankylosing spondylitis or reactive arthritis (a form of arthritis that occurs following infection in another part of the body, usually the genitourinary tract).

Treatment

Treatment for low back pain generally depends on whether the pain is acute or chronic. In general, surgery is recommended only if there is evidence of worsening nerve damage and when diagnostic tests indicate structural changes for which corrective surgical procedures have been developed.

Conventionally used treatments and their level of supportive evidence include:

Hot or cold packs have never been proven to quickly resolve low back injury; however, they may help ease pain and reduce inflammation for people with acute, subacute, or chronic pain, allowing for greater mobility among some individuals.

Activity: Bed rest should be limited. Individuals should begin stretching exercises and resume normal daily activities as soon as possible, while avoiding movements that aggravate pain. Strong evidence shows that persons who continue their activities without bed rest following onset of low back pain appeared to have better back flexibility than those who rested in bed for a week. Other studies suggest that bed rest alone may make back pain worse and can lead to secondary complications such as depression, decreased muscle tone, and blood clots in the legs.

Strengthening exercises, beyond general daily activities, are not advised for acute low back pain, but may be an effective way to speed recovery from chronic or subacute low back pain. Maintaining and building muscle strength is particularly important for persons with skeletal irregularities. Health care providers can provide a list of beneficial exercises that will help improve coordination and develop proper posture and muscle balance. Evidence supports short- and long-term benefits of yoga to ease chronic low back pain.

Physical therapy programs to strengthen core muscle groups that support the low back, improve mobility and flexibility, and promote proper positioning and posture are often used in combinations with other interventions.

Medications: A wide range of medications are used to treat acute and chronic low back pain. Some are available over the counter (OTC); others require a physician's prescription. Certain drugs, even those available OTC, may be unsafe during pregnancy, may interact with other medications, cause side effects, or lead to serious adverse effects such as liver damage or gastrointestinal ulcers and bleeding. Consultation with a health care provider is advised before use. The following are the main types of medications used for low back pain:

Analgesic medications are those specifically designed to relieve pain. They include OTC acetaminophen and aspirin, as well as prescription opioids such as codeine, oxycodone, hydrocodone, and morphine. Opioids should be used only for a short period of time and under a physician's supervision. People can develop a tolerance to opioids and require increasingly higher dosages to achieve the same effect. Opioids can also be addictive. Their side effects can include drowsiness, constipation, decreased reaction time, and impaired judgment. Some specialists are concerned that chronic use of opioids is detrimental to people with back pain because they can aggravate depression, leading to a worsening of the pain.

Nonsteroidal anti-inflammatory drugs (NSAIDS) relieve pain and inflammation and include OTC formulations (ibuprofen, ketoprofen, and naproxen sodium). Several others, including a type of NSAID called COX-2 inhibitors, are available only by prescription. Long-term use of NSAIDs has been associated with stomach irritation, ulcers, heartburn, diarrhea, fluid retention, and in rare cases, kidney dysfunction and cardiovascular disease. The longer a person uses NSAIDs the more likely they are to develop side effects. Many other drugs cannot be taken at the same time a person is treated with NSAIDs because they alter the way the body processes or eliminates other medications.

Anticonvulsants—drugs primarily used to treat seizures—may be useful in treating people with radiculopathy and radicular pain.

Antidepressants such as tricyclics and serotonin and norepinephrine reuptake inhibitors have been commonly prescribed for chronic low back pain, but their benefit for nonspecific low back pain is unproven, according to a review of studies assessing their benefit.

Counter-irritants such as creams or sprays applied topically stimulate the nerves in the skin to provide feelings of warmth or cold in order to dull the sensation of pain. Topical analgesics reduce inflammation and stimulate blood flow.

Spinal manipulation and spinal mobilization are approaches in which professionally licensed specialists (doctors of chiropractic care) use their hands to mobilize, adjust, massage, or stimulate the spine and the surrounding tissues. Manipulation involves a rapid movement over which the individual has no control; mobilization involves slower adjustment movements. The techniques have been shown to provide small to moderate short-term benefits in people with chronic low back pain. Evidence supporting their use for acute or subacute low back pain is generally of low quality. Neither technique is appropriate when a person has an underlying medical cause for the back pain such as osteoporosis, spinal cord compression, or arthritis.

Traction involves the use of weights and pulleys to apply constant or intermittent force to gradually "pull" the skeletal structure into better alignment. Some people experience pain relief while in traction, but that relief is usually temporary. Once traction is released the back pain tends to return. There is no evidence that traction provides any longterm benefits for people with low back pain.

Acupuncture is moderately effective for chronic low back pain. It involves the insertion of thin needles into precise points throughout the body. Some practitioners believe this process helps clear away blockages in the body's life force known as Qi (pronounced chee). Others who may not believe in the concept of Qi theorize that when the needles are inserted and then stimulated (by twisting or passing a low-voltage electrical current through them) naturally occurring painkilling chemicals such as endorphins, serotonin, and acetylcholine are released. Evidence of acupuncture's benefit for acute low back pain is conflicting and clinical studies continue to investigate its benefits.

Biofeedback is used to treat many acute pain problems, most notably back pain and headache. The therapy involves the attachment of electrodes to the skin and the use of an electromyography machine that allows people to become aware of and selfregulate their breathing, muscle tension, heart rate, and skin temperature. People regulate their response to pain by using relaxation techniques. Biofeedback is often used in combination with other treatment methods, generally without side effects. Evidence is lacking that biofeedback provides a clear benefit for low back pain.

Nerve block therapies aim to relieve chronic pain by blocking nerve conduction from specific areas of the body. Nerve block approaches range from injections of local anesthetics, botulinum toxin, or steroids into affected soft tissues or joints to more complex nerve root blocks and spinal cord stimulation. When extreme pain is involved, low doses of drugs may be administered by catheter directly into the spinal cord. The success of a nerve block approach depends on the ability of a practitioner to locate and inject precisely the correct nerve. Chronic use of steroid injections may lead to increased functional impairment.

Epidural steroid injections are a commonly used short-term option for treating low back pain and sciatica associated with inflammation. Pain relief associated with the injections, however, tends to be temporary and the injections are not advised for long-term use. An NIH-funded randomized controlled trial assessing the benefit of epidural steroid injections for the treatment of chronic low back pain associated with spinal stenosis showed that long-term outcomes were worse among those people who received the injections compared with those who did not.

Transcutaneous electrical nerve stimulation (TENS) involves wearing a battery-powered device consisting of electrodes placed on the skin over the painful area that generate electrical impulses designed to block incoming pain signals from the peripheral nerves. The theory is that stimulating the nervous system can modify the perception of pain. Early studies of TENS suggested that it elevated levels of endorphins, the body's natural pain-numbing chemicals. More recent studies, however, have produced mixed results on its effectiveness for providing relief from low back pain.

When other therapies fail, surgery may be considered an option to relieve pain caused by serious musculoskeletal injuries or nerve compression. It may be months following surgery before the patient is fully healed, and he or she may suffer permanent loss of flexibility.

Surgical procedures are not always successful, and there is little evidence to show which procedures work best for their particular indications. Patients considering surgical approaches should be fully informed of all related risks.

Prevention

Recurring back pain resulting from improper body mechanics is often preventable by avoiding movements that jolt or strain the back, maintaining correct posture, and lifting objects properly. Many work-related injuries are caused or aggravated by stressors such as heavy lifting, contact stress (repeated or constant contact between soft body tissue and a hard or sharp object), vibration, repetitive motion, and awkward posture. Using ergonomically designed furniture and equipment to protect the body from injury at home and in the workplace may reduce the risk of back injury.

The use of lumbar supports in the form of wide elastic bands that can be tightened to provide support to the lower back and abdominal muscles to prevent low back pain remains controversial. Such supports are widely used despite a lack of evidence showing that they actually prevent pain. Multiple studies have determined that the use of lumbar supports provides no benefit in terms of the prevention and treatment of back pain. Although there have been anecdotal case reports of injury reduction among workers using lumbar support belts, many companies that have back belt programs also have training and ergonomic awareness programs. The reported injury reduction may be related to a combination of these or other factors. Furthermore, some caution is advised given that wearing supportive belts may actually lead to or aggravate back pain by causing back muscles to weaken from lack of use.

Following any period of prolonged inactivity, a regimen of low-impact exercises is advised. Speed walking, swimming, or stationary bike riding 30 minutes daily can increase muscle strength and flexibility. Yoga also can help stretch and strengthen muscles and improve posture. Consult a physician for a list of low-impact, age-appropriate exercises that are specifically targeted to strengthening lower back and abdominal muscles.

Always stretch before exercise or other strenuous physical activity.

Don't slouch when standing or sitting. The lower back can support a person's weight most easily when the curvature is reduced. When standing, keep your weight balanced on your feet.

At home or work, make sure work surfaces are at a comfortable height.

Sit in a chair with good lumbar support and proper position and height for the task. Keep shoulders back. Switch sitting positions often and periodically walk around the office or gently stretch muscles to relieve tension. A pillow or rolled-up towel placed behind the small of the back can provide some lumbar support. During prolonged periods of sitting, elevate feet on a low stool or a stack of books.

Wear comfortable, low-heeled shoes.

Sleeping on one's side with the knees drawn up in a fetal position can help open up the joints in the spine and relieve pressure by reducing the curvature of the spine. Always sleep on a firm surface.

Don't try to lift objects that are too heavy. Lift from the knees, pull the stomach muscles in, and keep the head down and in line with a straight back. When lifting, keep objects close to the body. Do not twist when lifting.

Maintain proper nutrition and diet to reduce and prevent excessive weight gain, especially weight around the waistline that taxes lower back muscles. A diet with sufficient daily intake of calcium, phosphorus, and vitamin D helps to promote new bone growth.

Quit smoking. Smoking reduces blood flow to the lower spine, which can contribute to spinal disc degeneration. Smoking also increases the risk of osteoporosis and impedes healing. Coughing due to heavy smoking also may cause back pain.

(Source: National Institute of Neurological Disorders and Stroke, National Institutes of Health, Bethesda, MD [Feb 2015])

OSTEOPOROSIS

Among the bone diseases that afflict Americans, osteoporosis is by far the most prevalent. Patients with osteoporosis have thinned bones that result in bone fragility and an increased risk of fractures. In the United States, women are four times as likely to develop osteoporosis as men. The major fracture sites associated with osteoporosis are the hip, the spine, and the wrist. Of all injury sites, hip fractures have the greatest morbidity and socioeconomic impact. In the six months following hip fracture, there is an overall 12 to 20 percent reduction in expected survival, and 15 to 20 percent of patients will need to enter a long-term care institution shortly after the fracture.

Osteoporosis often goes undetected at first. Sometimes there are obvious signs that a person has osteoporosis — they may "shrink" a little and develop a stooped posture, for example. But often the first sign that someone has osteoporosis is when they break a bone, sometimes without knowing how or why it happened. This kind of break is called a "spontaneous fracture."

It is normal for your bones to become less dense as you grow older, but osteoporosis speeds up this process. This condition can particularly lead to problems in older age because broken bones do not heal as easily in older people as they do in young people, and the consequences are more serious. In general, osteoporosis is more common in women, and they often develop it at a younger age.

Getting older does not mean that you will automatically develop osteoporosis, but the risk does increase with age. People over the age of 70 are more likely to have low bone density. Plus, the risk of falling increases in old age, which then also makes fractures more likely.

But there are several things you can do to protect and strengthen your bones – even if you are already older.

Risk Factors

There are a number of factors that can increase someone's risk of developing osteoporosis. Some can be influenced, whereas others cannot. The main risk factors for osteoporosis include:

- Age: As we get older, our bone density decreases and the risk of developing osteoporosis increases. Men over the age of 65 and post-menopausal women are at the greatest risk.

- Sex: Women develop osteoporosis more often than men, and they are also more likely to have bone fractures.
- Low body weight (compared to body size)
- Diet low in calcium
- Vitamin D deficiency
- Lack of exercise
- Family history: Women whose mother or father broke their hip because of osteoporosis are at greater risk of developing osteoporosis themselves.
- Smoking
- Drinking a lot of alcohol
- Long-term steroid use
- Use of other medications, such as some antidepressants (SSRIs) or diabetes medicines (glitazones)
- Conditions such as rheumatoid arthritis or hyperthyroidism (an overactive thyroid gland)

Prevention

There are several things you can do on your own to protect your bones and lower your individual risk of developing osteoporosis. These include eating a diet rich in calcium, getting regular exercise and quitting smoking. Making sure your body has enough vitamin D is also important. Dietary supplements can be used as an additional source of calcium and vitamin D if you are not getting enough in your diet.

Femoral neck fractures are especially likely to have serious consequences because most people do not fully recover afterwards. Although osteoporosis can increase the likelihood of this kind of fracture, falls are the greatest risk factor for hip fractures. So it is especially important for older people to try to prevent falls. Getting exercise can help here: Physical activity can make you feel more confident and improve your coordination. It is also important to take care of hazards around your home that could increase your chances of slipping or stumbling. These may include things like loose cables, rugs and door thresholds.

Treatment

Osteoporosis can be treated with several drugs designed to slow bone loss and increase the production of new bone tissue. These include bisphosphonates and some hormonal or hormone-like medications. These kinds of drugs can have different types of side effects, though, and may not be suitable for everyone. They are only considered if someone has already broken a bone, or if their risk of bone fractures is high – for example, if their bone density is very low or if they have a combination of different risk factors, like low body weight, old age and a higher risk of falling.

Hormone products, like those used to treat menopause symptoms, can also lower the risk of osteoporosis-related bone fractures when taken over the long term. But long-term hormone therapy during or after menopause increases the risk of cardiovascular diseases and breast cancer. For this reason it is only rarely recommended as treatment for osteoporosis. The pros and cons of this treatment should be carefully weighed.

Research

A great many research efforts into osteoporosis are underway at the NIH. Fourteen institutes, centers, and divisions at the NIH support basic and/or clinical research on osteoporosis and related bone diseases. Much of the research is done collaboratively; both within the NIH and with agencies and organizations outside the NIH and outside the Federal Government. Studies being conducted range from investigations of the causes and consequences of bone loss at cellular and tissue levels to clinical trials testing strategies to maintain and even enhance bone density. Evaluation of skeletal status is of major concern as scientists explore the roles of such factors as anabolic hormones, calcium, vitamin D, drugs, and exercise on bone mass. The influence of environmental factors (e.g., cadmium lead, boron) is also being examined. Some scientists are investigating bone matrix formation and the effects of mechanical strain; others are assessing the regulation of osteoblasts (bone-forming cells) and osteoclasts (bone degrading cells). Numerous studies are focusing on various aspects of fractures, including identification of risk factors; associated with racial differences, as well as development of treatment interventions. Researchers are also looking at osteoporosis in men, the influence of alcohol on bone mineral density, and the abnormal development of cartilage. The association between osteoporosis and lupus is being explored, and a recently established bone clinic at the NIH is facilitating the development of diagnostic and treatment protocols.

All of these activities contribute to advancing science in this area, and have been made possible by recent breakthroughs in areas such as genetics and the development of cell lines and of osteoporosis-prone mouse models. Another recent advance—ultrasound measurements of bone offers a faster, cheaper and radiation-free alternative to other measures of bone density. This valuable new technology will help to identify those patients at a higher risk for fracture and will facilitate the targeting of individuals for preventive therapy. Exciting therapeutic avenues being pursued include the use of slow-release sodium fluoride, parathyroid hormone, and recombinant growth factors.

The Basic Osteoporosis: New Experimental Strategies (BONES) Initiative is an excellent example of a comprehensive NIH research approach that incorporates many different aspects of osteoporosis research. The goals of this initiative are to 1) encourage established bone biology investigators to address osteoporosis-related problems with novel approaches and the most powerful methodologies available; 2) increase the pool of investigators working in osteoporosis-related basic science areas by drawing researchers from genetics, cell and molecular biology, and structural chemistry into bone research; and 3) foster the development of interactions among laboratories originating in different disciplines.

Another NIH initiative investigates the remodeling (renewal) and repair of bone and connective tissue after damage from injury or degenerative disease. Natural repair is often insufficient, resulting in improper fracture healing, the failure of wounds to heal, and persistent joint dysfunction. This new initiative will look at a variety of factors that influence the tissue repair process, including how materials produced by cells affect the repair process, which cell populations are responsible for the repair and how these cells perform their functions, and whether techniques can be developed that would enable us to facilitate the repair processes.

Several clinical studies have also been launched to learn more about this crippling disorder. For example, one clinical trial seeks to determine the complementary and synergistic effects of exercise and hormone replacement on bone density and bone loss in postmenopausal women. Another clinical study is examining ways to correct calcium deficiency in young women thereby helping to prevent the likelihood of osteoporotic fractures later in life. In other efforts, a study of fluoride exposure and fractures has been initiated to learn more about the positive effect of slow-release fluoride in decreasing vertebral fractures in osteoporotic women.

The future is ripe with opportunities to build on recent progress. The previously-cited BONES and remodeling initiatives should yield important knowledge with regard to bone and connective tissue repair. Continued basic research into the molecular mechanisms of hormone action will provide additional insight into the causes and consequences of osteoporosis and related bone diseases. Clinical trials will be conducted with a goal of reducing the morbidity and mortality associated with these diseases. Human models and markers of skeletal aging are being developed. More functional prosthetic and orthotic devices will be designed, and additional outcomes of medical rehabilitation interventions will be measured. With every increment in knowledge, researchers will be better able to combat the devastating effects of bone diseases.

MUSCULAR DISORDERS

Muscular dystrophy is but one of many degenerative muscular disorders that cause tremendous suffering. Muscular dystrophy is an inherited muscle disorder in which there is slow but progressive wasting of muscle. Although there are several forms of muscular dystrophy, the most common is known as Duchenne muscular dystrophy. With this type, infants are slow in their ability to sit up and walk. When they do, it is with difficulty. Degeneration of the skeletal muscles that control movement proceeds rapidly. Eventually, the lung muscles become affected, leading to respiratory failure. Duchenne muscular dystrophy results from a defect in the gene that codes for a membrane-associated muscle protein called dystrophia. There is considerable support for research into understanding the function of this protein and for the utilization of muscle cells in gene therapy for correction of this disorder in humans.

There is no cure for muscular dystrophy. Treatments can help with the symptoms and prevent complications. They include physical and speech therapy, orthopedic devices, surgery, and medications. Some people with MD have mild cases that worsen slowly. Others cases are disabling and severe.

Drug therapy includes corticosteroids to slow muscle degeneration, anticonvulsants to control seizures and some muscle activity, immunosuppressants to delay some damage to dying muscle cells, and antibiotics to fight respiratory infections. Some individuals may benefit from occupational therapy and assistive technology. Some patients may need assisted ventilation to treat respiratory muscle weakness and a pacemaker for cardiac abnormalities.

SKIN DISEASES

The NIH also supports research into the causes and treatment of many types of disabling skin diseases. For example, epidermolysis bullosa represents 20 different forms of rare, hereditary blistering disorders that involve the skin and mucous membranes. Epidermolysis bullosa can range from a relatively mild condition to a severely disabling and sometimes fatal disease. The skin of patients with epidermolysis bullosa is extremely fragile, and the slightest friction can cause painful blistering. In severe or dystrophic epidermolysis bullosa, blisters can cover most of the body and occur in the digestive tract. Often wounds from severe epidermolysis bullosa resemble serious bums. Epidermolysis bullosa is a life-long disorder and can cause extreme physical, emotional, and financial hardships for the afflicted patients and their families. Researchers have identified the precise location in skin that is affected by epidermolysis bullosa and the genes that are mutated in the various forms of these diseases. Research results such as these continue to shed light on the genetic origin of the various forms of epidermolysis bullosa and have generated a renewed optimism for altering the course and for improving treatments for these diseases.

MULTIFACETED APPROACHES TO PREVENTING DISABILITY

Chronic disability is sometimes caused by a single injury or disease process, but for many individuals, particularly older persons, disability is the result of multiple, complex, and interacting factors. In addition to basic and clinical research to prevent and treat chronic diseases, successful new strategies now being developed and tested can make a critical contribution to quality of life and help prevent the disability that leads to long-term care. These strategies determine major risk factors for a specific disability, or disabling condition or event, based on epidemiologic research, and develop interventions for each major treatable risk factor. They then apply interventions to each individual on the basis of his or her specific risk factors, using simple, inexpensive technologies to prevent complex, expensive problems.

These interventions targeted risk factors for falls, such as bone fragility and muscle weakness, postural hypotension, use of sedatives or multiple medications, impairments of motion such as balance and gait, and environmental hazards. Participants receive individualized treatment, including medication adjustments, strength and balance training, and instruction on safe practices to avoid lightheadedness and environmental hazards. As a result of the interventions, participants' rate of falls was reduced by nearly half. Since more than 250,000 hip fractures occur each year among persons over age 65, a substantial national cost savings should result from incorporating the tested strategy into the usual health care of older persons.

Research on risk factors can also be applied to predicting disability. One such study of older nondisabled persons found that three short tests of physical performance abilities strongly predicted disability as much as four years in advance. Combining this knowledge with interventions such as the multiple risk factor approach has the potential of preventing or delaying onset of diseases such as diabetes and arthritis, disorders such as urinary incontinence and mobility impairments, adverse drug effects, and -nursing home admission. The potential impact on associated health care expenditures is estimated in tens of billions of dollars.

Researchers are identifying the behaviors that place individuals at greater risk for poor health, depression, and other negative outcomes. The well-documented benefits for health and longevity that come as a result of adopting healthy lifestyle practices, such as physical activity and nutrition, and terminating health impairing habits, such as smoking, apply at all ages, even to the very old. A large research portfolio is dedicated to find ways to overcome the impediments that can prevent people from initiating and maintaining health-enhancing behaviors or adhering to medical regimens that can extend the healthy years of life.

Investigators are also monitoring the nation's disability rates. Studies have shown that these rates were significantly lower in older people than those predicted by prior analyses. Research is underway to determine the causes underlying the decline and to apply this information where possible to reducing disability.

One of the most exciting research frontiers involves the examination of the interaction among behavior, central nervous system structure and function, and neuroendocrine and other hormonal factors. Care givers of persons with chronic disabling diseases have been found to be prone to negative health outcomes because of the stresses inherent in the often difficult aspects of caregiving. Research promises to develop effective interventions to help alleviate the burdens of long-term care for care givers.

11

Vaccination and Immunization

Vaccines are the best defense we have against serious, preventable, and sometimes deadly contagious diseases. Vaccines are some of the safest medical products available, but like any other medical product, there may be risks. Accurate information about the value of vaccines as well as their possible side-effects helps people to make informed decisions about vaccination.

Understanding the difference between vaccines, vaccinations, and immunizations can be tricky. Below is an easy guide that explains how these terms are used:

A vaccine is a product that produces immunity from a disease and can be administered through needle injections, by mouth, or by aerosol.

A vaccination is the injection of a killed or weakened organism that produces immunity in the body against that organism.

An immunization is the process by which a person or animal becomes protected from a disease. Vaccines cause immunization, and there are also some diseases that cause immunization after an individual recovers from the disease.

Many partners work together to make sure vaccines are safe. Government health scientists work with manufacturers, health care providers, academia, and global health groups such as the World Health Organization to offer a comprehensive vaccine safety system. At the Department of Health and Human Services, primarily three agencies are involved in vaccine safety:

Centers for Disease Control and Prevention (CDC)

Food and Drug Administration (FDA)

National Institutes of Health (NIH)

Vaccines are held to the highest standard of safety. The United States currently has the safest, most effective vaccine supply in history. Vaccines undergo extensive testing and rigorous evaluation by FDA and are approved only after FDA has determined that the scientific information supports safety and effectiveness.   Once a vaccine is approved, FDA regularly inspects vaccine manufacturing facilities to make sure strict regulations are followed.   Vaccines are manufactured in batches called lots and vaccine manufacturers must test all lots of a vaccine to ensure safety, purity, and potency.   Vaccine lots cannot be distributed to the public until released by FDA.

Scientists from FDA and CDC work closely to monitor reports of vaccine side effects (adverse events) after they are approved and used widely. FDA and CDC take all reports seriously, and work together to evaluate and address any potential problems.

Federal law requires that Vaccine Information Statements explaining vaccine benefits and risks be provided when certain vaccinations are administered (before each dose). Vaccine Information Statements are available in Spanish and many different languages. In addition, more detailed information describing the benefits and risks of vaccines is available in the Prescribing Information from the Food and Drug Administration.

VACCINES FOR CHILDREN

Currently, CDC recommends vaccination against 16 vaccine preventable diseases for children.

Vaccines are our best defense against many diseases, which often result in serious complications such as pneumonia, meningitis (swelling of the lining of the brain), liver cancer, bloodstream infections, and even death. CDC recommends vaccinations to protect children against 16 infectious diseases, including measles, mumps, rubella (German measles), varicella (chickenpox), hepatitis B, diphtheria, tetanus, pertussis (whooping cough), Haemophilus influenza type B (Hib), polio, influenza (flu), and pneumococcal disease.

Children are given vaccines at a young age because this is when they are most vulnerable to certain diseases. Newborn babies are immune to some diseases because they have antibodies given to them from their mothers. However, this immunity only lasts a few months. Further, most young children do not have maternal immunity to diphtheria, whooping cough, polio, tetanus, hepatitis B, or Hib. If a child is not vaccinated and is exposed to a disease, the child's body may not be strong enough to fight the disease.

An infant's immune system is more than ready to respond to the very small number of weakened and killed infectious agents (antigens) in vaccines. From the time they are born, babies are exposed to thousands of germs and other antigens in the environment and their immune systems are readily able to respond to these large numbers of antigenic stimuli.

A combination vaccine consists of two or more different vaccines that have been combined into a single shot. Combination vaccines have been in use in the United States since the mid-1940's. Examples of combination vaccines in current use are: DTaP (diphtheria-tetanus-pertussis), trivalent IPV (three strains of inactivated polio vaccine), MMR (measles-mumps-rubella), DTaP-Hib, and Hib-Hep B (hepatitis B). Simultaneous vaccination is when more than one vaccine shot is administered during the same doctor's visit, usually in separate limbs (e.g. one in each arm). An example of simultaneous vaccination might be administering DTap in one arm or leg and IPV in another arm or leg during the same visit.

Giving a child several vaccinations during the same visit offers two practical advantages. First, we want to immunize children as quickly as possible to give them protection during the vulnerable early months of their lives. Second, giving several vaccinations at the same time means fewer office visits. This saves parents both time and money, and may be less traumatic for the child.

The available scientific data show that simultaneous vaccination with multiple vaccines has no adverse effect on the normal childhood immune system. A number of studies have been conducted to examine the effects of giving various combinations of vaccines simultaneously. These studies have shown that the recommended vaccines are as effective in combination as they are individually, and that such combinations carry no greater risk for adverse side effects. Consequently, both the Advisory Committee on Immunization Practices and the American Academy of Pediatrics recommend simultaneous administration of all routine childhood vaccines when appropriate. Research is underway to find methods to combine more antigens in a single vaccine injection (for example, MMR and chickenpox).

No evidence suggests that the recommended childhood vaccines can "overload" the immune system. In contrast, from the moment babies are born, they are exposed to numerous bacteria and viruses on a daily basis. Eating food introduces new bacteria into the body; numerous bacteria live in the mouth and nose; and an infant places his or her hands or other objects in his or her mouth hundreds of times every hour, exposing the immune system to still more antigens. When a child has a cold they are exposed to at least 4 to 10 antigens and exposure to "strep throat" is about 25 to 50 antigens.

Sometimes, fevers can cause a person to experience spasms or jerky movements called seizures. These seizures related to fever are called febrile seizures. Febrile seizures can happen with any condition that causes a fever. Causes include common childhood illnesses like colds, the flu, an ear infection, or roseola. Vaccines sometimes cause fevers, but febrile seizures are rare after vaccination.

Up to 5% of young children will have at least one febrile seizure, usually associated with getting sick. Most febrile seizures happen in children between the ages of 6 months and 5 years. The most common age range to have a febrile seizure is 14–18 months. The recommended age for the first doses of MMRV, MMR, and varicella vaccines is 12-14 months old. During this time children in this age group are recommended to receive other routine vaccines as well.

Getting a child vaccinated as soon as recommended prevents febrile seizures by protecting young children against measles, mumps, rubella, chickenpox, influenza, pneumococcal infections and other diseases that can cause fever and febrile seizures.

During a febrile seizure, a child often has spasms or jerking movements and may lose consciousness. Febrile seizures usually last one or two minutes, and they do not cause any permanent neurological damage. They are most common with fevers of 102°F (38.9°C) or higher, but they can also happen at lower body temperatures or when a fever is going down.

Febrile seizures can be frightening, but nearly all children who have a febrile seizure recover quickly and are healthy afterwards. About 1 in 3 children who have one febrile seizure will have at least one more during childhood; some of these are linked to family health history. There is a small increased risk for febrile seizures after MMR and MMRV vaccines.

Studies have shown a small increased risk for febrile seizures during the first to second week after the first vaccination with measles, mumps, rubella (MMR) vaccine and the first dose of measles, mumps, rubella, and varicella (MMRV) vaccine. Studies have not shown an increased risk for febrile seizures after the acellular pertussis vaccine, DTaP, or after varicella (chickenpox) vaccine.

One vaccine called DTP (whole cell pertussis), which is no longer used in the United States, had a small increased risk for febrile seizures after DTP on the day the vaccine was given.

Vaccines and Autism

There is no link between vaccines and autism. Some people have had concerns that Autism might be linked to the vaccines children receive, but studies have shown that there is no link between receiving vaccines and developing Autism.

One vaccine ingredient that has been studied specifically is thimerosal, a mercury-based preservative used to prevent contamination of multidose vials of vaccines. Research shows that thimerosal does not cause Autism. In fact, a 2004 scientific review by the IOM concluded that "the evidence favors rejection of a causal relationship between thimerosal–containing vaccines and autism." Since 2003, there have been nine CDC-funded or conducted studies that have found no link between thimerosal-containing vaccines and Autism, as well as no link between the measles, mumps, and rubella (MMR) vaccine and Autism in children.

Between 1999 and 2001, thimerosal was removed or reduced to trace amounts in all childhood vaccines except for some flu vaccines. This was done as part of a broader national effort to reduce all types of mercury exposure in children before studies were conducted that determined that thimerosal was not harmful.   It was done as a precaution. Currently, the only childhood vaccines that contain thimerosal are flu vaccines packaged in multidose vials. Thimerosal-free alternatives are also available for flu vaccine.*

EFFECTIVENESS

Vaccines work really well. Of course, no medicine is perfect but most childhood vaccines produce immunity about 90 - 100% of the time. Better hygiene and sanitation can help prevent the spread of disease, but the germs that cause disease will still be around. As long as germs still exist, they will continue to make people sick. If you look at the history of any vaccine-preventable disease, you will virtually always see that the number of cases of disease starts to drop when a vaccine is licensed.

The measles vaccine was licensed in 1962, and that's when the number of cases started to decline. If the drop in disease were due to hygiene and sanitation, you would expect all diseases to start going away at about the

---

* http://www.cdc.gov/vaccinesafety/Concerns/Autism/Index.html

same time. But if you were to look at the figures for polio, for example, you would see the number of cases start to drop around 1955 – the year the first polio vaccine was licensed. If you look at the figures for Hib, the number drops around 1990, for pneumococcal disease around 2000 — corresponding to the introduction of vaccines for those diseases.

Vaccines are the most effective tool we have to prevent infectious diseases.*

PREVENTION AND PROTECTION

Infections are the most common cause of human disease. Disease-causing microbes (pathogens) attempting to get into the body must move past the body's external armor, usually the skin or cells lining the body's internal passageways, and your immune system if these microbes get inside.   Your immune system works because is able to tell if an invader (virus, bacteria, parasite, or other another person's tissues) has entered it— even if you aren't consciously aware that anything has happened. Your body recognizes this invader and uses a number of different tactics to destroy it.

Vaccines help the body's immune system prepare for future attacks. Vaccines consist of killed or modified microbes, parts of microbes, or microbial DNA that trick the body into thinking an infection has occurred.   A vaccinated person's immune system attacks the harmless vaccine and prepares for invasions against the kind of microbe the vaccine contained. In this way, the person becomes immunized against the microbe: if re-exposure to the infectious microbe occurs, the immune system will quickly recognize how to stop the infection.

When a critical portion of a community is immunized against a contagious disease, most members of the community are protected against that disease because there is little opportunity for an outbreak. Even those who are not eligible for certain vaccines—such as infants, pregnant women, or immunocompromised individuals—get some protection because the spread of contagious disease is contained. This is known as "community immunity."

The principle of community immunity applies to control of a variety of contagious diseases, including influenza, measles, mumps, rotavirus, and pneumococcal disease.

---

* http://www.vaccines.gov/basics/effectiveness/index.html

Knowing which vaccines you need is an important step toward protecting your health and that of your family and friends.   Getting vaccines on time helps prevent illness before you're exposed.

If you are sick, you may still be able to receive a vaccine, depending on which vaccine you need and the type and severity of your illness. Talk with your health care provider about the vaccines that might be recommended for your age, health status, and lifestyle.

Vaccine schedules are designed with you in mind.   They are constructed to be as safe and as convenient as possible, without requiring unnecessary visits to your doctor or health care provider.

Infants, Children, & Teens (birth to age 18)

Vaccinating your child is one of the most important steps you can take to protect their health and future. The childhood vaccine schedule designed to be as safe and as convenient as possible, and to protect children when they are at highest risk of complications from disease. Help protect your child's health by learning about the vaccines they need and being sure to get the pre-teen and teenage vaccines on time. If your child did not get these vaccines at age 11 or 12, schedule an appointment to get them now. Vaccines are an important part of preventive care throughout life.

Child Catch-up (age 4 months to 18 years)

If your child is behind on his or her vaccines, don't worry – they can get caught up on all the recommended vaccines at any age.   Some schools and child care centers may require your child to be up-to-date on certain recommended vaccines before entrance. Speak with your doctor to learn how to get your child safely back on track.

Schedule

Hepatitis B (HepB) vaccine.
Routine vaccination: At birth:
Doses following the birth dose:
The second dose should be administered at age 1 or 2 months. Monovalent HepB vaccine should be used for doses administered before age 6 weeks.

Administration of a total of 4 doses of HepB vaccine is permitted when a combination vaccine containing HepB is administered after the birth dose.

Catch-up vaccination:

Unvaccinated persons should complete a 3-dose series.

A 2-dose series (doses separated by at least 4 months) of adult formulation Recombivax HB is licensed for use in children aged 11 through 15 years.

Rotavirus (RV) vaccines.

Minimum age: 6 weeks for both RV1 [Rotarix] and RV5 [RotaTeq])

Routine vaccination: Administer a series of RV vaccine to all infants as follows:

If Rotarix is used, administer a 2-dose series at 2 and 4 months of age.

If RotaTeq is used, administer a 3-dose series at ages 2, 4, and 6 months.

If any dose in the series was RotaTeq or vaccine product is unknown for any dose in the series, a total of 3 doses of RV vaccine should be administered.

Catch-up vaccination:

The maximum age for the first dose in the series is 14 weeks, 6 days; vaccination should not be initiated for infants aged 15 weeks, 0 days or older.

The maximum age for the final dose in the series is 8 months, 0 days.

Diphtheria and tetanus toxoids and acellular pertussis (DTaP) vaccine.

Minimum age: 6 weeks. Exception: DTaP-IPV [Kinrix]: 4 years)

Routine vaccination:

Administer a 5-dose series of DTaP vaccine at ages 2, 4, 6, 15 through 18 months, and 4 through 6 years. The fourth dose may be administered as early as age 12 months, provided at least 6 months have elapsed since the third dose. However, the fourth dose of DTaP need not be repeated if it was administered at least 4 months after the third dose of DTaP.

Catch-up vaccination:

The fifth dose of DTaP vaccine is not necessary if the fourth dose was administered at age 4 years or older.

Tetanus and diphtheria toxoids and acellular pertussis (Tdap) vaccine.

Minimum age: 10 years for both Boostrix and Adacel)

Routine vaccination:

Administer 1 dose of Tdap vaccine to all adolescents aged 11 through 12 years.

Tdap may be administered regardless of the interval since the last tetanus and diphtheria toxoid-containing vaccine.

Administer 1 dose of Tdap vaccine to pregnant adolescents during each pregnancy (preferred during 27 through 36 weeks' gestation) regardless of time since prior Td or Tdap vaccination.

Catch-up vaccination:

Persons aged 7 years and older who are not fully immunized with DTaP vaccine should receive Tdap vaccine as 1 dose (preferably the first) in the catch-up series; if additional doses are needed, use Td vaccine. For children 7 through 10 years who receive a dose of Tdap as part of the catch-up series, an adolescent Tdap vaccine dose at age 11 through 12 years should NOT be administered. Td should be administered instead 10 years after the Tdap dose.

Persons aged 11 through 18 years who have not received Tdap vaccine should receive a dose followed by tetanus and diphtheria toxoid (Td) booster doses every 10 years thereafter.

Inadvertent doses of DTaP vaccine:

If administered inadvertently to a child aged 7 through 10 years may count as part of the catch-up series. This dose may count as the adolescent Tdap dose, or the child can later receive a Tdap booster dose at age 11 through 12 years.

If administered inadvertently to an adolescent aged 11 through 18 years, the dose should be counted as the adolescent Tdap booster.

Haemophilus influenzae type b (Hib) conjugate vaccine.

Minimum age: 6 weeks for PRP-T [ACTHIB, DTaP-IPV/Hib (Pentacel) and Hib-MenCY (MenHibrix)], PRP-OMP [PedvaxHIB or COMVAX], 12 months for PRP-T [Hiberix])

Routine vaccination:

Administer a 2- or 3-dose Hib vaccine primary series and a booster dose (dose 3 or 4 depending on vaccine used in primary series) at age 12 through 15 months to complete a full Hib vaccine series.

The primary series with ActHIB, MenHibrix, or Pentacel consists of 3 doses and should be administered at 2, 4, and 6 months of age. The primary series with PedvaxHib or COMVAX consists of 2 doses and should be administered at 2 and 4 months of age; a dose at age 6 months is not indicated.

One booster dose (dose 3 or 4 depending on vaccine used in primary series) of any Hib vaccine should be administered at age 12 through 15 months. An exception is Hiberix vaccine. Hiberix should only be used for the booster (final) dose in children aged 12 months through 4 years who have received at least 1 prior dose of Hib-containing vaccine.

Catch-up vaccination:

If dose 1 was administered at ages 12 through 14 months, administer a second (final) dose at least 8 weeks after dose 1, regardless of Hib vaccine used in the primary series.

If both doses were PRP-OMP (PedvaxHIB or COMVAX), and were administered before the first birthday, the third (and final) dose should be administered at age 12 through 59 months and at least 8 weeks after the second dose.

If the first dose was administered at age 7 through 11 months, administer the second dose at least 4 weeks later and a third (and final) dose at age 12 through 15 months or 8 weeks after second dose, whichever is later.

If first dose is administered before the first birthday and second dose administered at younger than 15 months, a third (and final) dose should be given 8 weeks later.

For unvaccinated children aged 15 months or older, administer only 1 dose.

Vaccination of persons with high-risk conditions:

Children aged 12 through 59 months who are at increased risk for Hib disease, including chemotherapy recipients and those with anatomic or functional asplenia (including sickle cell disease), human immunodeficiency virus (HIV) infection, immunoglobulin deficiency, or early component complement deficiency, who have received either no doses or only 1 dose of Hib vaccine before 12 months of age, should receive 2 additional doses of Hib vaccine 8 weeks apart; children who received 2 or more doses of Hib vaccine before 12 months of age should receive 1 additional dose.

For patients younger than 5 years of age undergoing chemotherapy or radiation treatment who received a Hib vaccine dose(s) within 14 days of starting therapy or during therapy, repeat the dose(s) at least 3 months following therapy completion.

Recipients of hematopoietic stem cell transplant (HSCT) should be revaccinated with a 3-dose regimen of Hib vaccine starting 6 to 12 months after successful transplant, regardless of vaccination history; doses should be administered at least 4 weeks apart.

A single dose of any Hib-containing vaccine should be administered to unimmunized* children and adolescents 15 months of age and older undergoing an elective splenectomy; if possible, vaccine should be administered at least 14 days before procedure.

Hib vaccine is not routinely recommended for patients 5 years or older. However, 1 dose of Hib vaccine should be administered to unimmunized* persons aged 5 years or older who have anatomic or functional asplenia (including sickle cell disease) and unvaccinated persons 5 through 18 years of age with human immunodeficiency virus (HIV) infection.

* Patients who have not received a primary series and booster dose or at least 1 dose of Hib vaccine after 14 months of age are considered unimmunized.

Pneumococcal vaccines.

Minimum age: 6 weeks for PCV13, 2 years for PPSV23)

Routine vaccination with PCV13:

Administer a 4-dose series of PCV13 vaccine at ages 2, 4, and 6 months and at age 12 through 15 months.

For children ages 14 through 59 months who have received an age-appropriate series of 7-valent PCV (PCV7), administer a single supplemental dose of 13-valent PCV (PCV13).

Catch-up vaccination with PCV13:

Administer 1 dose of PCV13 to all healthy children aged 24 through 59 months who are not completely vaccinated for their age.

Inactivated poliovirus vaccine (IPV).

Minimum age: 6 weeks)

Routine vaccination:

Administer a 4-dose series of IPV at ages 2, 4, 6 through 18 months, and 4 through 6 years. The final dose in the series should be administered on or after the fourth birthday and at least 6 months after the previous dose.

Catch-up vaccination:

In the first 6 months of life, minimum age and minimum intervals are only recommended if the person is at risk for imminent exposure to circulating poliovirus (i.e., travel to a polio-endemic region or during an outbreak).

If 4 or more doses are administered before age 4 years, an additional dose should be administered at age 4 through 6 years and at least 6 months after the previous dose.

A fourth dose is not necessary if the third dose was administered at age 4 years or older and at least 6 months after the previous dose.

If both OPV and IPV were administered as part of a series, a total of 4 doses should be administered, regardless of the child's current age. IPV is not routinely recommended for U.S. residents aged 18 years or older.

Influenza vaccines.

Minimum age: 6 months for inactivated influenza vaccine [IIV], 2 years for live, attenuated influenza vaccine [LAIV])

Routine vaccination:

Administer influenza vaccine annually to all children beginning at age 6 months. For most healthy, nonpregnant persons aged 2 through 49 years, either LAIV or IIV may be used. However, LAIV should NOT be administered to some persons, including 1) persons who have experienced severe allergic reactions to LAIV, any of its components, or to a previous dose of any other influenza vaccine; 2) children 2 through 17 years receiving aspirin or aspirin-containing products; 3) persons who are allergic to eggs; 4) pregnant women; 5) immunosuppressed persons; 6) children 2 through 4 years of age with asthma or who had wheezing in the past 12 months; or 7) persons who have taken influenza antiviral medications in the previous 48 hours.

For children aged 6 months through 8 years:

For the 2015–16 season, follow dosing guidelines in the 2015 ACIP influenza vaccine recommendations.

For persons aged 9 years and older:

Administer 1 dose.

Measles, mumps, and rubella (MMR) vaccine.

Minimum age: 12 months for routine vaccination)

Routine vaccination:

Administer a 2-dose series of MMR vaccine at ages 12 through 15 months and 4 through 6 years. The second dose may be administered before age 4 years, provided at least 4 weeks have elapsed since the first dose.

Administer 1 dose of MMR vaccine to infants aged 6 through 11 months before departure from the United States for international travel. These children should be revaccinated with 2 doses of MMR vaccine, the first at age 12 through 15 months (12 months if the child remains in an area where disease risk is high), and the second dose at least 4 weeks later.

Administer 2 doses of MMR vaccine to children aged 12 months and older before departure from the United States for international travel. The first dose should be administered on or after age 12 months and the second dose at least 4 weeks later.

Catch-up vaccination:

Ensure that all school-aged children and adolescents have had 2 doses of MMR vaccine; the minimum interval between the 2 doses is 4 weeks.

Varicella (VAR) vaccine.

Minimum age: 12 months)

Routine vaccination:

Administer a 2-dose series of VAR vaccine at ages 12 through 15 months and 4 through 6 years. The second dose may be administered before age 4 years, provided at least 3 months have elapsed since the first dose. If the second dose was administered at least 4 weeks after the first dose, it can be accepted as valid.

Catch-up vaccination:

Ensure that all persons aged 7 through 18 years without evidence of immunity have two doses of varicella vaccine. For children aged 7 through 12 years, the recommended minimum interval between doses is 3 months (if the second dose was administered at least 4 weeks after the first dose, it can be accepted as valid); for persons aged 13 years and older, the minimum interval between doses is 4 weeks.

Hepatitis A (HepA) vaccine.

Minimum age: 12 months)

Routine vaccination:

Initiate the 2-dose HepA vaccine series at 12 through 23 months; separate the 2 doses by 6 to 18 months.

Children who have received 1 dose of HepA vaccine before age 24 months should receive a second dose 6 to 18 months after the first dose.

For any person aged 2 years and older who has not already received the HepA vaccine series, 2 doses of HepA vaccine separated by 6 to 18 months may be administered if immunity against hepatitis A virus infection is desired.

Catch-up vaccination:

The minimum interval between the two doses is 6 months.

Special populations:

Administer 2 doses of HepA vaccine at least 6 months apart to previously unvaccinated persons who live in areas where vaccination programs target older children, or who are at increased risk for infection. This includes persons traveling to or working in countries that have high or intermediate endemicity of infection; men having sex with men; users of injection and non-injection illicit drugs; persons who work with HAV-infected primates or with HAV in a research laboratory; persons with clotting-factor disorders; persons with chronic liver disease; and persons who anticipate close personal contact (e.g., household or regular babysitting) with an international adoptee during the first 60 days after arrival in the United States from a country with high or intermediate endemicity. The first dose should be administered as soon as the adoption is planned, ideally 2 or more weeks before the arrival of the adoptee.

Human papillomavirus (HPV) vaccines.

Minimum age: 9 years for HPV2 [Cervarix] and HPV4 [Gardasil])

Routine vaccination:

Administer a 3-dose series of HPV vaccine on a schedule of 0, 1-2, and 6 months to all adolescents aged 11 through 12 years. Either HPV4 or HPV2 may be used for females, and only HPV4 may be used for males.

The vaccine series may be started at age 9 years.

Administer the second dose 1 to 2 months after the first dose (minimum interval of 4 weeks); administer the third dose 24 weeks after the first dose and 16 weeks after the second dose (minimum interval of 12 weeks).

Catch-up vaccination:

Administer the vaccine series to females (either HPV2 or HPV4) and males (HPV4) at age 13 through 18 years if not previously vaccinated.

Use recommended routine dosing intervals (see above) for vaccine series catch-up.

Meningococcal conjugate vaccines.

Minimum age: 6 weeks for Hib-MenCY [MenHibrix], 9 months for MenACWY-D [Menactra], 2 months for MenACWY-CRM [Menveo])

Routine vaccination:

Administer a single dose of Menactra or Menveo vaccine at age 11 through 12 years, with a booster dose at age 16 years.

Adolescents aged 11 through 18 years with human immunodeficiency virus (HIV) infection should receive a 2-dose primary series of Menactra or Menveo with at least 8 weeks between doses.

For children aged 2 months through 18 years with high-risk conditions, see below.

Catch-up vaccination:

Administer Menactra or Menveo vaccine at age 13 through 18 years if not previously vaccinated.

If the first dose is administered at age 13 through 15 years, a booster dose should be administered at age 16 through 18 years with a minimum interval of at least 8 weeks between doses.

If the first dose is administered at age 16 years or older, a booster dose is not needed.

Vaccination of persons with high-risk conditions and other persons at increased risk of disease:

Children with anatomic or functional asplenia (including sickle cell disease):

Menveo

Children who initiate vaccination at 8 weeks through 6 months: Administer doses at 2, 4, 6, and 12 months of age.

Unvaccinated children 7 through 23 months: Administer 2 doses, with the second dose at least 12 weeks after the first dose AND after the first birthday.

Children 24 months and older who have not received a complete series: Administer 2 primary doses at least 8 weeks apart.

MenHibrix

Children 6 weeks through 18 months: Administer doses at 2, 4, 6, and 12 through 15 months of age.

If the first dose of MenHibrix is given at or after 12 months of age, a total of 2 doses should be given at least 8 weeks apart to ensure protection against serogroups C and Y meningococcal disease.

Menactra

Children 24 months and older who have not received a complete series: Administer 2 primary doses at least 8 weeks apart. If Menactra is administered to a child with asplenia (including sickle cell disease), do not administer Menactra until 2 years of age and at least 4 weeks after the completion of all PCV13 doses.

Children with persistent complement component deficiency:

Menveo

Children who initiate vaccination at 8 weeks through 6 months: Administer doses at 2, 4, 6 and 12 months of age.

Unvaccinated children 7 through 23 months: Administer two doses, with the second dose at least 12 weeks after the first dose AND after the first birthday.

Children 24 months and older who have not received a complete series: Administer 2 primary doses at least 8 weeks apart.

MenHibrix

Children 6 weeks through 18 months: Administer doses at 2, 4, 6, and 12 through 15 months of age.

If the first dose of MenHibrix is given at or after 12 months of age, a total of 2 doses should be given at least 8 weeks apart to ensure protection against serogroups C and Y meningococcal disease.

Menactra

Children 9 through 23 months; Administer 2 primary doses at least 12 weeks apart.

Children 24 months and older who have not received a complete series: Administer 2 primary doses at least 8 weeks apart.

For children who travel to or reside in countries in which meningococcal disease is hyperendemic or epidemic, including countries in the African meningitis belt or the Hajj, administer an age- appropriate formulation and series of Menactra or Menveo for protection against serogroups A and W meningococcal disease. Prior receipt of MenHibrix is not sufficient for children traveling to the meningitis belt or the Hajj because it does not contain serogroups A or W.

For children at risk during a community outbreak attributable to a vaccine serogroup, administer or complete an age- and formulation-appropriate series of MenHibrix, Menactra, or Menveo.

College & Young Adults (age 19 to 24)

Young adulthood often means increased independence, changes, and responsibilities.   Most vaccines are given early in childhood, but college students, armed services recruits, and young adults need certain immunizations, too. Learn more about the vaccines are specifically recommended for young adults ages 19-24.

Most vaccines are given early in childhood, but college students and young adults need certain immunizations, too.   These vaccines are specifically recommended for young adults ages 19-24:

- Meningococcal conjugate vaccine protects against bacterial meningitis and may be required for some college freshmen or other students living in a dorm.
- Tdap vaccine protects against tetanus, diphtheria, and pertussis, or whooping cough.
- HPV vaccine protects against the human papillomavirus (HPV), which causes most cases of cervical and anal cancers, as well as genital warts.
- Seasonal flu vaccine.

Adults (age 19 and older)

Immunizations are not just for kids!   Whether a college student, middle-aged adult, or senior citizen, all adults need immunizations to keep them and their families healthy.

Influenza vaccination

Annual vaccination against influenza is recommended for all persons aged 6 months or older.

Persons aged 6 months or older, including pregnant women and persons with hives-only allergy to eggs can receive the inactivated influenza vaccine (IIV). An age-appropriate IIV formulation should be used.

Adults aged 18 years or older can receive the recombinant influenza vaccine (RIV) (FluBlok). RIV does not contain any egg protein and can be given to age-appropriate persons with egg allergy of any severity.

Healthy, nonpregnant persons aged 2 to 49 years without high-risk medical conditions can receive either intranasally administered live, attenuated influenza vaccine (LAIV) (FluMist) or IIV.

Health care personnel who care for severely immunocompromised persons who require care in a protected environment should receive IIV or RIV; health care personnel who receive LAIV should avoid providing care for severely immunosuppressed persons for 7 days after vaccination.

The intramuscularly or intradermally administered IIV are options for adults aged 18 through 64 years.

Adults aged 65 years or older can receive the standard-dose IIV or the high-dose IIV (Fluzone High-Dose).

Tetanus, diphtheria, and acellular pertussis (Td/Tdap) vaccination

Administer 1 dose of Tdap vaccine to pregnant women during each pregnancy (preferably during 27 to 36 weeks' gestation) regardless of interval since prior Td or Tdap vaccination.

Persons aged 11 years or older who have not received Tdap vaccine or for whom vaccine status is unknown should receive a dose of Tdap followed by tetanus and diphtheria toxoids (Td) booster doses every 10 years thereafter. Tdap can be administered regardless of interval since the most recent tetanus or diphtheria-toxoid containing vaccine.

Adults with an unknown or incomplete history of completing a 3-dose primary vaccination series with Td-containing vaccines should begin or complete a primary vaccination series including a Tdap dose.

For unvaccinated adults, administer the first 2 doses at least 4 weeks apart and the third dose 6 to 12 months after the second.

For incompletely vaccinated (i.e., less than 3 doses) adults, administer remaining doses.

Varicella vaccination

All adults without evidence of immunity to varicella (as defined below) should receive 2 doses of single-antigen varicella vaccine or a second dose if they have received only 1 dose.

Vaccination should be emphasized for those who have close contact with persons at high risk for severe disease (e.g., health care personnel and family contacts of persons with immunocompromising conditions) or are at high risk for exposure or transmission (e.g., teachers; child care employees; residents and staff members of institutional settings, including correctional institutions; college students; military personnel; adolescents and adults living in households with children; nonpregnant women of childbearing age; and international travelers).

Pregnant women should be assessed for evidence of varicella immunity. Women who do not have evidence of immunity should receive the first dose of varicella vaccine upon completion or termination of pregnancy and before discharge from the health care facility. The second dose should be administered 4 to 8 weeks after the first dose.

Evidence of immunity to varicella in adults includes any of the following: documentation of 2 doses of varicella vaccine at least 4 weeks apart;

U.S.-born before 1980, except health care personnel and pregnant women;

history of varicella based on diagnosis or verification of varicella disease by a health care provider;

history of herpes zoster based on diagnosis or verification of herpes zoster disease by a health care provider; or

laboratory evidence of immunity or laboratory confirmation of disease.

Human papillomavirus (HPV) vaccination

Two vaccines are licensed for use in females, bivalent HPV vaccine (HPV2) and quadrivalent HPV vaccine (HPV4), and one HPV vaccine for use in males (HPV4).

For females, either HPV4 or HPV2 is recommended in a 3-dose series for routine vaccination at age 11 or 12 years and for those aged 13 through 26 years, if not previously vaccinated.

For males, HPV4 is recommended in a 3-dose series for routine vaccination at age 11 or 12 years and for those aged 13 through 21 years, if not previously vaccinated. Males aged 22 through 26 years may be vaccinated.

HPV4 is recommended for men who have sex with men through age 26 years for those who did not get any or all doses when they were younger.

Vaccination is recommended for immunocompromised persons (including those with HIV infection) through age 26 years for those who did not get any or all doses when they were younger.

A complete series for either HPV4 or HPV2 consists of 3 doses. The second dose should be administered 4 to 8 weeks (minimum interval of 4 weeks) after the first dose; the third dose should be administered 24 weeks after the first dose and 16 weeks after the second dose (minimum interval of at least 12 weeks).

HPV vaccines are not recommended for use in pregnant women. However, pregnancy testing is not needed before vaccination. If a woman is found to be pregnant after initiating the vaccination series, no intervention is needed; the remainder of the 3-dose series should be delayed until completion or termination of pregnancy.

Zoster vaccination

A single dose of zoster vaccine is recommended for adults aged 60 years or older regardless of whether they report a prior episode of herpes zoster. Although the vaccine is licensed by the U.S. Food and Drug Administration for use among and can be administered to persons aged 50 years or older, ACIP recommends that vaccination begin at age 60 years.

Persons aged 60 years or older with chronic medical conditions may be vaccinated unless their condition constitutes a contraindication, such as pregnancy or severe immunodeficiency.

Measles, mumps, rubella (MMR) vaccination

Adults born before 1957 are generally considered immune to measles and mumps. All adults born in 1957 or later should have documentation of 1 or more doses of MMR vaccine unless they have a medical contraindication to the vaccine or laboratory evidence of immunity to each of the three diseases. Documentation of provider-diagnosed disease is not considered acceptable evidence of immunity for measles, mumps, or rubella.

Measles component:

A routine second dose of MMR vaccine, administered a minimum of 28 days after the first dose, is recommended for adults who:

are students in postsecondary educational institutions,

work in a health care facility, or

plan to travel internationally.

Persons who received inactivated (killed) measles vaccine or measles vaccine of unknown type during 1963–1967 should be revaccinated with 2 doses of MMR vaccine.

Mumps component:

A routine second dose of MMR vaccine, administered a minimum of 28 days after the first dose, is recommended for adults who:

are students in a postsecondary educational institution,

work in a health care facility, or

plan to travel internationally.

Persons vaccinated before 1979 with either killed mumps vaccine or mumps vaccine of unknown type who are at high risk for mumps infection (e.g., persons who are working in a health care facility) should be considered for revaccination with 2 doses of MMR vaccine.

Rubella component:

For women of childbearing age, regardless of birth year, rubella immunity should be determined. If there is no evidence of immunity, women who are not pregnant should be vaccinated. Pregnant women who do not have evidence of immunity should receive MMR vaccine upon completion or termination of pregnancy and before discharge from the health care facility.

Pneumococcal (13-valent pneumococcal conjugate vaccine [PCV13] and 23-valent pneumococcal polysaccharide vaccine [PPSV23]) vaccination
General information
When indicated, only a single dose of PCV13 is recommended for adults.

No additional dose of PPSV23 is indicated for adults vaccinated with PPSV23 at or after age 65 years.

When both PCV13 and PPSV23 are indicated, PCV13 should be administered first; PCV13 and PPSV23 should not be administered during the same visit.

When indicated, PCV13 and PPSV23 should be administered to adults whose pneumococcal vaccination history is incomplete or unknown.

Adults aged 65 years or older who
Have not received PCV13 or PPSV23: Administer PCV13 followed by PPSV23 in 6 to 12 months.

Have not received PCV13 but have received a dose of PPSV23 at age 65 years or older: Administer PCV13 at least 1 year after the dose of PPSV23 received at age 65 years or older.

Have not received PCV13 but have received 1 or more doses of PPSV23 before age 65: Administer PCV13 at least 1 year after the most recent dose of PPSV23; administer a dose of PPSV23 6 to 12 months after PCV13, or as soon as possible if this time window has passed, and at least 5 years after the most recent dose of PPSV23.

Have received PCV13 but not PPSV23 before age 65 years: Administer PPSV23 6 to 12 months after PCV13 or as soon as possible if this time window has passed.

Have received PCV13 and 1 or more doses of PPSV23 before age 65 years: Administer PPSV23 6 to 12 months after PCV13, or as soon as possible if this time window has passed, and at least 5 years after the most recent dose of PPSV23.

Adults aged 19 through 64 years with immunocompromising conditions or anatomical or functional asplenia (defined below) who
Have not received PCV13 or PPSV23: Administer PCV13 followed by PPSV23 at least 8 weeks after PCV13; administer a second dose of PPSV23 at least 5 years after the first dose of PPSV23.

Have not received PCV13 but have received 1 dose of PPSV23: Administer PCV13 at least 1 year after the PPSV23; administer a second dose of PPSV23 at least 8 weeks after PCV13 and at least 5 years after the first dose of PPSV23.

Have not received PCV13 but have received 2 doses of PPSV23: Administer PCV13 at least 1 year after the most recent dose of PPSV23.

Have received PCV13 but not PPSV23: Administer PPSV23 at least 8 weeks after PCV13; administer a second dose of PPSV23 at least 5 years after the first dose of PPSV23.

Have received PCV13 and 1 dose of PPSV23: Administer a second dose of PPSV23 at least 5 years after the first dose of PPSV23.

Adults aged 19 through 64 years with cerebrospinal fluid leaks or cochlear implants: Administer PCV13 followed by PPSV23 at least 8 weeks after PCV13.

Adults aged 19 through 64 years with chronic heart disease (including congestive heart failure and cardiomyopathies, excluding hypertension), chronic lung disease (including chronic obstructive lung disease, emphysema, and asthma), chronic liver disease (including cirrhosis), alcoholism, or diabetes mellitus: Administer PPSV23.

Adults aged 19 through 64 years who smoke cigarettes or reside in nursing home or long-term care facilities: Administer PPSV23.

Routine pneumococcal vaccination is not recommended for American Indian/Alaska Native or other adults unless they have the indications as above; however, public health authorities may consider recommending the use of pneumococcal vaccines for American Indians/Alaska Natives or other adults who live in areas with increased risk for invasive pneumococcal disease.

Immunocompromising conditions that are indications for pneumococcal vaccination are: congenital or acquired immunodeficiency (including B- or T-lymphocyte deficiency, complement deficiencies, and phagocytic disorders excluding chronic granulomatous disease), HIV infection, chronic renal failure, nephrotic syndrome, leukemia, lymphoma, Hodgkin disease, generalized malignancy, multiple myeloma, solid organ transplant, and iatrogenic immunosuppression (including long-term systemic corticosteroids and radiation therapy).

Anatomical or functional asplenia that are indications for pneumococcal vaccination are: sickle cell disease and other hemoglobinopathies, congenital or acquired asplenia, splenic dysfunction, and splenectomy. Administer pneumococcal vaccines at least 2 weeks before immunosuppressive therapy or an elective splenectomy, and as soon as possible to adults who are newly diagnosed with asymptomatic or symptomatic HIV infection.

Meningococcal vaccination

Administer 2 doses of quadrivalent meningococcal conjugate vaccine (MenACWY [Menactra, Menveo]) at least 2 months apart to adults of all ages with anatomical or functional asplenia or persistent complement component deficiencies. HIV infection is not an indication for routine vaccination with MenACWY. If an HIV-infected person of any age is vaccinated, 2 doses of MenACWY should be administered at least 2 months apart.

Administer a single dose of meningococcal vaccine to microbiologists routinely exposed to isolates of Neisseria meningitidis, military recruits, persons at risk during an outbreak attributable to a vaccine serogroup, and persons who travel to or live in countries in which meningococcal disease is hyperendemic or epidemic.

First-year college students up through age 21 years who are living in residence halls should be vaccinated if they have not received a dose on or after their 16th birthday.

MenACWY is preferred for adults with any of the preceding indications who are aged 55 years or younger as well as for adults aged 56 years or older who a) were vaccinated previously with MenACWY and are recommended for revaccination, or b) for whom multiple doses are anticipated. Meningococcal polysaccharide vaccine (MPSV4 [Menomune]) is preferred for adults aged 56 years or older who have not received MenACWY previously and who require a single dose only (e.g., travelers).

Revaccination with MenACWY every 5 years is recommended for adults previously vaccinated with MenACWY or MPSV4 who remain at increased risk for infection (e.g., adults with anatomical or functional asplenia, persistent complement component deficiencies, or microbiologists).

Hepatitis A vaccination

Vaccinate any person seeking protection from hepatitis A virus (HAV) infection and persons with any of the following indications:

men who have sex with men and persons who use injection or noninjection illicit drugs;

persons working with HAV-infected primates or with HAV in a research laboratory setting;

persons with chronic liver disease and persons who receive clotting factor concentrates;

persons traveling to or working in countries that have high or intermediate endemicity of hepatitis A; and

unvaccinated persons who anticipate close personal contact (e.g., household or regular babysitting) with an international adoptee during the first 60 days after arrival in the United States from a country with high or intermediate endemicity. The first dose of the 2-dose hepatitis A vaccine series should be administered as soon as adoption is planned, ideally 2 or more weeks before the arrival of the adoptee.

Single-antigen vaccine formulations should be administered in a 2-dose schedule at either 0 and 6 to 12 months (Havrix), or 0 and 6 to 18 months (Vaqta). If the combined hepatitis A and hepatitis B vaccine (Twinrix) is used, administer 3 doses at 0, 1, and 6 months; alternatively, a 4-dose schedule may be used, administered on days 0, 7, and 21 to 30 followed by a booster dose at month 12.

Hepatitis B vaccination

Vaccinate persons with any of the following indications and any person seeking protection from hepatitis B virus (HBV) infection:

sexually active persons who are not in a long-term, mutually monogamous relationship (e.g., persons with more than 1 sex partner during the previous 6 months); persons seeking evaluation or treatment for a sexually transmitted disease (STD); current or recent injection drug users; and men who have sex with men;

health care personnel and public safety workers who are potentially exposed to blood or other infectious body fluids;

persons with diabetes who are younger than age 60 years as soon as feasible after diagnosis; persons with diabetes who are age 60 years or older at the discretion of the treating clinician based on the likelihood of acquiring HBV infection, including the risk posed by an increased need for assisted blood glucose monitoring in long-term care facilities, the likelihood of experiencing chronic sequelae if infected with HBV, and the likelihood of immune response to vaccination;

persons with end-stage renal disease, including patients receiving hemodialysis, persons with HIV infection, and persons with chronic liver disease;

household contacts and sex partners of hepatitis B surface antigen–positive persons, clients and staff members of institutions for persons with developmental disabilities, and international travelers to countries with high or intermediate prevalence of chronic HBV infection; and

all adults in the following settings: STD treatment facilities, HIV testing and treatment facilities, facilities providing drug abuse treatment and prevention services, health care settings targeting services to injection drug users or men who have sex with men, correctional facilities, end-stage renal disease programs and facilities for chronic hemodialysis patients, and institutions and nonresidential day care facilities for persons with developmental disabilities.

Administer missing doses to complete a 3-dose series of hepatitis B vaccine to those persons not vaccinated or not completely vaccinated. The second dose should be administered 1 month after the first dose; the third dose should be given at least 2 months after the second dose (and at least 4 months after the first dose). If the combined hepatitis A and hepatitis B vaccine (Twinrix) is used, give 3 doses at 0, 1, and 6 months; alternatively, a 4-dose Twinrix schedule, administered on days 0, 7, and 21 to 30 followed by a booster dose at month 12 may be used.

Adult patients receiving hemodialysis or with other immunocompromising conditions should receive 1 dose of 40 mcg/mL (Recombivax HB) administered on a 3-dose schedule at 0, 1, and 6 months or 2 doses of 20 mcg/mL (Engerix-B) administered simultaneously on a 4-dose schedule at 0, 1, 2, and 6 months.

Haemophilus influenzae type b (Hib) vaccination

One dose of Hib vaccine should be administered to persons who have anatomical or functional asplenia or sickle cell disease or are undergoing elective splenectomy if they have not previously received Hib vaccine. Hib vaccination 14 or more days before splenectomy is suggested.

Recipients of a hematopoietic stem cell transplant (HSCT) should be vaccinated with a 3-dose regimen 6 to 12 months after a successful transplant, regardless of vaccination history; at least 4 weeks should separate doses.

Hib vaccine is not recommended for adults with HIV infection since their risk for Hib infection is low.

Immunocompromising conditions

Inactivated vaccines generally are acceptable (e.g., pneumococcal, meningococcal, and inactivated influenza vaccine) and live vaccines generally are avoided in persons with immune deficiencies or immunocompromising conditions. See ACIP Recommendations for information on specific conditions.

Seniors (age 65 and older)

Vaccines for older adults can prevent serious diseases and even death. They can also help prevent the spread of disease through your family and community. You may need one or more vaccines, even if you received vaccines as a child or as a younger adult. Ask your doctor which ones are right for you. Vaccines recommended for older adults can prevent:

- Influenza (Flu)
- Shingles (Herpes Zoster)
- Diphtheria/Tetanus
- Pertussis (Whooping Cough)

- Pneumococcal (Pneumonia)

Pregnant

Vaccines can help keep you and your growing family healthy. If you are pregnant or planning a pregnancy, the specific vaccinations you need are determined by factors such as your age, lifestyle, high-risk conditions, type and locations of travel, and previous vaccinations.

Recommended before Pregnancy

Before becoming pregnant, you should be up-to-date on routine adult vaccines. This will help protect you and your child. Generally speaking, live vaccines should not be given within a month before conception, while inactivated (killed) vaccines may be given at any time before or during pregnancy, if needed. It is best to talk to your healthcare provider about vaccinations before you become pregnant.

Recommended during Pregnancy

It is safe and very important for a woman who is pregnant during flu season to receive the inactivated flu vaccine. A pregnant woman who gets the flu is at risk for serious complications and hospitalization. Pregnant woman with flu also have a greater chance for serious problems for their unborn baby, including premature labor and delivery.

It is also very safe and important for pregnant women to receive the whooping cough vaccine (Tdap). Whooping cough, or pertussis, can be life-threatening for infants. Vaccinating expectant mothers against whooping cough reduces the risk to her and her infant. Tdap is also recommended for others who spend time with infants.

Recommended after Pregnancy

It is safe for a woman to receive vaccines right after giving birth, even while she is breastfeeding. New mothers who have never received Tdap, should be vaccinated right after delivery. Also, a woman who is not immune to measles, mumps and rubella and/or varicella (chickenpox) should be vaccinated before leaving the hospital.

Did you know that your baby gets disease immunity (protection) from you during pregnancy? But this protection is temporary and only for the diseases that you are immune to.

VACCINATIONS FOR OVERSEAS TRAVEL

Some countries require foreign visitors to carry an International Certificate of Vaccination (aka Yellow Card) or other proof that they have had certain inoculations or medical tests before entering or transiting their country. Before you travel, check the Country Specific Information and contact the foreign embassy of the country to be visited or transited through for county entry requirements.

Be sure that you and your family are up to date on your routine vaccinations. These vaccines are necessary for protection from diseases that are still common in many parts of the world even though they rarely occur in the United States.

Recommended Vaccinations

These vaccines are recommended to protect travelers from illnesses present in other parts of the world and to prevent infectious diseases from crossing international borders. Which vaccinations you need will depend on a number of factors including your destination, whether you will be spending time in rural areas, the season of the year you are traveling, your age, health status, and previous immunizations.

Required Vaccinations

Currently, the only vaccine required by International Health Regulations is yellow fever vaccination for travel to certain countries in sub-Saharan Africa and tropical South America. Meningococcal vaccination is required by the government of Saudi Arabia for annual travel during the Hajj.

Even when it is not required, yellow fever vaccine may be highly recommended for persons traveling to countries within endemic zones. The vaccine is highly effective at preventing the disease. After primary immunization with a single injected dose, booster doses are needed at 10-year intervals. Vaccination with the yellow fever vaccine is valid 10 days after the primary dose and immediately after booster doses.

Cholera vaccine is no longer administered in the U.S. However, contrary to WHO regulations, proof of cholera vaccination may occasionally be required as a condition of entry into some countries. Some countries with cholera-infected areas may still require evidence of a full primary series and a current booster dose. Thus, travelers to cholera endemic areas should be advised to check with the appropriate embassies or consulates before departure, particularly if they anticipate travel between two countries with active cholera outbreaks.

To avoid cholera vaccination at a border (or even quarantine in some countries), travelers may need a physician's signed statement (on letterhead) that cholera vaccine is contraindicated because of underlying health conditions.

Your immunizations should be documented in an International Certificate of Vaccination (Yellow Card). It is a good idea to keep this Certificate with your passport so you don't misplace it. It is recognized internationally and may be required before entry to certain countries.

It is important to consult with a travel health specialist concerning immunizations that may be recommended for your destination and specific itinerary. It is critical to realize that the health and sanitation conditions for the country you are visiting are not the same as here in the U.S. Thanks to decades of public health initiatives in the United States, many contagious diseases have been eliminated. But when a traveler goes to a country that is not similarly protected, a person can be at dangerous risk of contracting a disease. The principle behind a vaccine or immunization is to expose your body's system to the disease after it has been rendered harmless. By doing so, the body can build up its own natural protection so that if it encounters the virus, the body will be "immune" to its effects. This immunization effect takes time, so it is a good idea to give your body at least a month head start to condition itself before traveling.

The Immunization Practices Advisory Committee of the Centers for Disease Control and Prevention (CDC) recommends that all persons be up-to-date on routine immunizations, regardless of travel plans. Outbreaks of measles, polio, and pertussis have occurred in developing countries where populations were inadequately immunized, and susceptible visitors have been stricken with travel-acquired measles and poliovirus infections.   There have now even been outbreaks of measles and pertussis in the U.S.

The primary series of tetanus, diphtheria, pertussis, MMR and polio vaccines is customarily given in childhood. Surveillance data suggests that a significant percentage of North Americans over the age of 20 do not update their tetanus/diphtheria immunizations at the recommended 10-year interval. Although polio boosters are not routinely given in North America, they are recommended before travel to known polio endemic and developing areas.

Other travel-related vaccines

Hepatitis A is an acute viral infection which produces loss of appetite, nausea, vomiting, fatigue, weakness, muscle pain, sore throat, jaundice and cough often lasting one to two weeks or more. It is spread by contaminated food, water, milk, shellfish and contact with persons who have the infection. No specific treatment is available. Protection from Hepatitis A infection requires a series of two doses of the Hepatitis A vaccine, six months apart.

Hepatitis B is a serious disease that affects the liver and can in some people lead to chronic infection, cirrhosis, liver cancer, and death.   It is spread by contact with blood or bodily fluids. The Hep B vaccine can prevent the disease and is recommended for all international travelers. The standard dosing regimen consists of three injections at 0, 1, and 6 months.

Japanese Encephalitis is a viral infection spread by infected mosquitoes in many areas of Southeast Asia and India. For those traveling to high-risk areas, vaccination is recommended.   Protection requires a two dose series, 28 days apart.

Meningococcal is caused by a bacterium that enters the body through the respiratory system. It is the leading cause of bacterial meningitis in young adults.   Meningitis is an infection of the fluid surrounding the brain and spinal cord.   Meningococcal is active in several countries throughout the world.   Protection is obtained through vaccination. There are two kinds of meningococcal vaccine available in the U.S. One is the preferred vaccine for people 2 through 55 years of age. The other is generally recommended for those older than 55.   A meningococcal vaccine is required who those who travel to the annual pilgrimage to Mecca (Hajj). Those travelers must be vaccinated at least 10 days before arriving to Saudi Arabia.

Typhoid fever is a serious bacterial disease which if not treated can kill up to 30% of people who get it.   It is normally contracted from contaminated food or water, although some people who get typhoid become "carriers" and spread the disease to others.   In areas where the disease is common avoid drinking the water and always practice good hygiene.

Yellow fever is a serious disease caused by yellow fever virus and spread through the bite of an infected mosquito. It is found in parts of Africa and

South America. Precautions and insect repellent are recommended to prevent exposure to yellow fever virus and include remaining in well-screened areas, wearing clothing that covers most of the body, and using effective insect repellent containing DEET. If traveling to endemic area, you should receive the yellow fever vaccine.

12

Communicable Illness

Chronic illnesses are not the only cause for strong public health concern in America, as a growing number of communicable illnesses have proven to be just as threatening to an individual's health. While research attempts to predict the future of health care needs, epidemics and pandemics of illness can strike without warning or proper preparation. In 2012, an outbreak of meningitis brought over 720 cases and 48 deaths, as well as a wave of West Nile Virus, which caused 243 deaths out of 5,387 cases.

In the 2014-15 flu season, the U.S. was exposed to a stronger strain of the influenza virus than ever before, and while a vaccine was available, it proved to be less effect with the elderly who have a higher mortality rate from effects of the virus.

Also last year the world watched in horror as the Ebola virus raced through several West African nations, killing up to 90 percent of those infected. It takes little imagination to think what might happen if several people with the Ebola virus – or any other deadly disease – were able to board a plane and travel undetected across the world.

According to a report by the National Intelligence Council "The dramatic increase in drug-resistant microbes, combined with the lag in development of new antibiotics, the rise of megacities with severe health care deficiencies, environmental degradation, and the growing ease and frequency of cross-border movements of people and produce have greatly facilitated the spread of infectious diseases."

Its conclusions were:

New and reemerging infectious diseases will pose a rising global health threat and will complicate US and global security over the next 20 years. These diseases will endanger US citizens at home and abroad, threaten US armed forces deployed overseas, and exacerbate social and political instability in key countries and regions in which the United States has significant interests.

Infectious diseases are a leading cause of death, accounting for a quarter to a third of the estimated 54 million deaths worldwide in 1998. The spread of infectious diseases results as much from changes in human behavior--including lifestyles and land use patterns, increased trade and travel, and inappropriate use of antibiotic drugs--as from mutations in pathogens.

Twenty well-known diseases--including tuberculosis (TB), malaria, and cholera--have reemerged or spread geographically since 1973, often in more virulent and drug-resistant forms.

At least 30 previously unknown disease agents have been identified since 1973, including HIV, Ebola, hepatitis C, and Nipah virus, for which no cures are available.

Of the seven biggest killers worldwide, TB, malaria, hepatitis, and, in particular, HIV/AIDS continue to surge, with HIV/AIDS and TB likely to account for the overwhelming majority of deaths from infectious diseases in developing countries by 2020. Acute lower respiratory infections--including pneumonia and influenza--as well as diarrheal diseases and measles, appear to have peaked at high incidence levels.

"Many infectious diseases--most recently, the West Nile virus--originate outside US borders and are introduced by international travelers, immigrants, returning US military personnel, or imported animals and foodstuffs. In the opinion of the US Institute of Medicine, the next major infectious disease threat to the United States may be, like HIV, a previously unrecognized pathogen. Barring that, the most dangerous known infectious diseases likely to threaten the United States over the next two decades will be HIV/AIDS, hepatitis C, TB, and new, more lethal variants of influenza. Hospital-acquired infections and foodborne illnesses also will pose a threat."

Discussing the implications for U.S. National Security, the report said: As a major hub of global travel, immigration, and commerce with wide-ranging interests and a large civilian and military presence overseas, the United States and its equities abroad will remain at risk from infectious diseases.

Emerging and reemerging infectious diseases, many of which are likely to continue to originate overseas, will continue to kill at least 170,000 Americans annually. Many more could perish in an epidemic of influenza or yet-unknown disease or if there is a substantial decline in the effectiveness of available HIV/AIDS drugs.

Infectious diseases are likely to continue to account for more military hospital admissions than battlefield injuries. US military personnel deployed at NATO and US bases overseas, will be at low-to-moderate risk. At highest risk will be US military forces deployed in support of humanitarian and peacekeeping operations in developing countries.

The infectious disease burden will weaken the military capabilities of some countries--as well as international peacekeeping efforts--as their armies and recruitment pools experience HIV infection rates ranging from 10 to 60 percent. The cost will be highest among officers and the more modernized militaries in Sub-Saharan Africa and increasingly among FSU states and possibly some rogue states.

Infectious diseases are likely to slow socioeconomic development in the hardest-hit developing and former communist countries and regions. This will challenge democratic development and transitions and possibly contribute to humanitarian emergencies and civil conflicts.

Infectious disease-related embargoes and restrictions on travel and immigration will cause frictions among and between developed and developing countries.

The probability of a bioterrorist attack against US civilian and military personnel overseas or in the United States also is likely to grow as more states and groups develop a biological warfare capability. Although there is no evidence that the recent West Nile virus outbreak in New York City was caused by foreign state or nonstate actors, the scare and several earlier instances of suspected bioterrorism showed the confusion and fear they can sow regardless of whether or not they are validated.

Infectious disease microbes are constantly evolving, oftentimes into new strains that are increasingly resistant to available antibiotics. As a result, an expanding number of strains of diseases--such as TB, malaria, and pneumonia--will remain difficult or virtually impossible to treat. At the same time, large-scale use of antibiotics in both humans and livestock will continue to encourage development of microbial resistance. The firstline drug treatment for malaria is no longer effective in over 80 of the 92 countries where the disease is a major health problem. Penicillin has substantially lost its effectiveness against several diseases, such as pneumonia, meningitis, and gonorrhea, in many countries. Eighty percent of Staphylococcus aureus isolates in the United States, for example, are penicillin-resistant and 32 percent are methicillin-resistant. A US Centers for Disease Control and Prevention (USCDC) study found a 60-fold increase in high-level resistance to penicillin among one group of Streptococcus pneumoniae cases in the United States and significant resistance to multidrug therapy as well. Influenza viruses, in particular, are particularly efficient in their ability to survive and genetically change, sometimes into deadly strains. HIV also displays a high rate of genetic mutation that will present significant problems in the development of an effective vaccine or new, affordable therapies.

EBOLA

The 2014 Ebola epidemic was the largest in history affecting multiple countries in West Africa. The U.S. sent medical personnel to assist, two of whom became affected and were airlifted back home – both survived. Two other infected people managed to enter the U.S. and both were hospitalized, one survived and the other died.

The Ebola virus causes an acute, serious illness which is often fatal if untreated. Ebola virus disease (EVD) first appeared in 1976 in 2 simultaneous outbreaks, one in Sudan, and the other in the Democratic Republic of Congo. The latter occurred in a village near the Ebola River, from which the disease takes its name.

The current outbreak in West Africa, (first cases notified in March 2014), is the largest and most complex Ebola outbreak since the Ebola virus was first discovered in 1976. There have been more cases and deaths in this outbreak than all others combined. It has also spread between countries starting in Guinea then spreading across land borders to Sierra Leone and Liberia, by air to Nigeria, and by land to Senegal.

The most severely affected countries, Guinea, Sierra Leone and Liberia have very weak health systems, lacking human and infrastructural resources, having only recently emerged from long periods of conflict

Transmission

It is thought that fruit bats are natural Ebola virus hosts. Ebola is introduced into the human population through close contact with the blood, secretions, organs or other bodily fluids of infected animals such as chimpanzees, gorillas, fruit bats, monkeys, forest antelope and porcupines found ill or dead or in the rainforest. Ebola then spreads through human-to-human transmission via direct contact (through broken skin or mucous membranes) with the blood, secretions, organs or other bodily fluids of infected people, and with surfaces and materials (e.g. bedding, clothing) contaminated with these fluids.

Health-care workers have frequently been infected while treating patients with suspected or confirmed EVD. This has occurred through close contact with patients when infection control precautions are not strictly practiced. Burial ceremonies in which mourners have direct contact with the body of the deceased person can also play a role in the transmission of Ebola.

People remain infectious as long as their blood and body fluids, including semen and breast milk, contain the virus. Men who have recovered from the disease can still transmit the virus through their semen for up to 7 weeks after recovery from illness.

Symptoms

The incubation period, that is, the time interval from infection with the virus to onset of symptoms is 2 to 21 days. Humans are not infectious until they develop symptoms. First symptoms are the sudden onset of fever fatigue, muscle pain, headache and sore throat. This is followed by vomiting, diarrhea, rash, symptoms of impaired kidney and liver function, and in some cases, both internal and external bleeding (e.g. oozing from the gums, blood in the stools). Laboratory findings include low white blood cell and platelet counts and elevated liver enzymes.

It can be difficult to distinguish EVD from other infectious diseases such as malaria, typhoid fever and meningitis. Confirmation that symptoms are caused by Ebola virus infection are made using the following investigations:
antibody-capture enzyme-linked immunosorbent assay (ELISA)
antigen-capture detection tests
serum neutralization test
reverse transcriptase polymerase chain reaction (RT-PCR) assay
electron microscopy
virus isolation by cell culture.
Samples from patients are an extreme biohazard risk; laboratory testing on non-inactivated samples should be conducted under maximum biological containment conditions.

Treatment

Supportive care-rehydration with oral or intravenous fluids- and treatment of specific symptoms, improves survival. There is as yet no proven treatment available for EVD. However, a range of potential treatments including blood products, immune therapies and drug therapies are currently being evaluated. No licensed vaccines are available yet, but 2 potential vaccines are undergoing human safety testing.

Good outbreak control relies on applying a package of interventions, namely case management, surveillance and contact tracing, a good laboratory service, safe burials and social mobilization. Community engagement is key to successfully controlling outbreaks. Raising awareness of risk factors for Ebola infection and protective measures that individuals can take is an effective way to reduce human transmission. Risk reduction messaging should focus on several factors:

Reducing the risk of wildlife-to-human transmission from contact with infected fruit bats or monkeys/apes and the consumption of their raw meat. Animals should be handled with gloves and other appropriate protective clothing. Animal products (blood and meat) should be thoroughly cooked before consumption.

Reducing the risk of human-to-human transmission from direct or close contact with people with Ebola symptoms, particularly with their bodily fluids. Gloves and appropriate personal protective equipment should be worn when taking care of ill patients at home. Regular hand washing is required after visiting patients in hospital, as well as after taking care of patients at home.

Outbreak containment measures including prompt and safe burial of the dead, identifying people who may have been in contact with someone infected with Ebola, monitoring the health of contacts for 21 days, the importance of separating the healthy from the sick to prevent further spread, the importance of good hygiene and maintaining a clean environment.

INFLUENZA

For more than a decade the World Health Organization (WHO) and other international agencies have warned that an influenza (flu) pandemic is both "inevitable" and "imminent." The warnings were originally issued because of concerns over avian (bird) flu, which emerged in Hong Kong in 1997. Over the next few years it spread throughout Asia, the Middle East and Europe; over half (56 percent) of the people affected died. It then re-emerged as a highly virulent strain of bird flu in the Middle East, Africa and Europe.

A more recent strain H7N9 in China was declared "one of the most lethal" of its kind, according to world health experts. It transmits more easily to humans and has already killed more than one in five of those affected.

"This is definitely one of the most lethal influenza viruses that we have seen so far," said Keiji Fukuda, the WHO's assistant director-general for health security. "When we look at influenza viruses, this is an unusually dangerous virus for humans," he said.

Some experts have called this strain a "super-flu" because scientists who analyzed genetic sequence data from samples from three H7N9 victims said it was a "triple reassortant" virus with a combination of genes from three other flu strains found in birds in Asia.

Recent pandemic viruses, including the H1N1 "swine flu" have been mixtures of mammal and bird flu - hybrids that are more likely to be milder because mammalian flu tends to make people less severely ill than bird flu. Pure bird flu strains, such as the new H7N9 strain and the H5N1 flu, which has killed about 371 of 622 of the people it has infected since 2003, are generally far more deadly for people.

Pandemics

Any animal influenza virus that develops the ability to infect people can theoretically cause a pandemic. Flu pandemics are global epidemics of a newly emerged strain of flu to which most people have little or no immunity. As a result they spread rapidly to affect most countries and regions around the world. While it is unlikely that a pandemic flu virus will originate in the United States, no country is exempt from risk. Once a pandemic virus emerges, we will probably not be able to prevent its global spread; but by being prepared we can significantly reduce its impact.

Much of our understanding of pandemic flu comes from the experience of three major flu pandemics last century, the first and worst of which in 1918 killed up to 40 million people worldwide—more lives lost than during the First World War. As history has shown, pandemic flu differs from "ordinary" flu in important ways.

For example, "ordinary" flu occurs seasonally, allowing us time to identify the virus and administer a vaccine in advance, whereas pandemic flu can occur at any time, allowing no time for a vaccine to be prepared because the virus is completely new. "Ordinary" flu most seriously affects the elderly and vulnerable groups, while pandemic flu can affect people of any age. These differences strongly influence the way in which we respond to pandemic flu.

Unlike the "ordinary" flu that occurs every winter, pandemic flu can occur at any time of year. Pandemics often come in two or more waves several months apart. Each wave may last two to three months. Pandemic flu is more serious than "ordinary" flu. Up to a quarter of the population can be affected—sometimes more. Pandemic flu is likely to cause the same symptoms as "ordinary" flu but the symptoms may be more severe because nobody has immunity or protection against a new virus.

A serious pandemic causes many deaths, disrupts the daily life of many people, and causes intense pressure on health and other services. Each pandemic is different, and until the virus starts circulating, it is impossible to predict its full effects. There is no vaccine ready to protect against pandemic flu. A vaccine cannot be made until the new virus has been identified. Before a pandemic starts it is difficult to predict what strain will cause it and even then, predictions may prove wrong. Also, the new virus may have changed enough for a pre-prepared vaccine to be ineffective. "Ordinary" flu vaccines will not protect against pandemic flu. But "ordinary" flu can be serious, so it is very important that everyone who is due an "ordinary" flu vaccine has one.

Prevention

You can reduce, but not eliminate, the risk of catching or spreading influenza during a pandemic by:
• Covering your nose and mouth when coughing or sneezing, using a tissue when possible
• Disposing of dirty tissues promptly and carefully
• Avoiding nonessential travel and large crowds whenever possible
• Maintaining good basic hygiene, for example washing your hands frequently with soap and water to reduce the spread of the virus from your hands to your face, or to other people
• Cleaning hard surfaces (e.g., kitchen counters, door handles) frequently using a normal cleaning product
• Making sure your children follow this advice

If you do catch flu:
• Stay at home and rest.
• Take medicines such as aspirin, ibuprofen, or paracetamol to relieve the symptoms (following the instructions with the medicines).
• Children under sixteen must not be given aspirin or ready-made flu remedies containing aspirin.

• Drink plenty of fluids

Experts predict anything between two million and fifty million deaths globally from the next pandemic.

During the pandemics of 1957 and 1968, the viruses took only three to four months to spread from southeast Asia—where they were first identified—to Europe and North America. The intercontinental spread of Severe Acute Respiratory Syndrome (SARS) in 2003 was even faster (see below). Within four months of the global alert, more than eight thousand people had been affected in thirty countries across six continents, and nine hundred people had died. The expansion of international air travel is likely to make the spread of pandemic flu just as rapid.

Ordinary Flu versus Avian Flu

Flu is an illness resulting from infection by an influenza virus. It is highly infectious and can spread easily from person to person. Because the flu virus constantly changes there are many different strains of flu. Some are more infectious and cause more severe illness than others.

People are affected by flu with varying degrees of severity, ranging from minor symptoms to pneumonia and death. Symptoms are generally of sudden onset and include:
• Fever
• Cough
• Headache
• Severe weakness and fatigue
• Aching muscles and joints
• Sore throat
• Runny nose

The symptoms of pandemic flu are similar to "ordinary" seasonal flu. However, in the case of pandemic flu, these symptoms are likely to be worse, resulting in more severe illness and possibly death.

Flu viruses are divided into three main groups: influenza A, B, and C. Type A viruses are the source of most "ordinary" flu epidemics and have caused all previous pandemics. Whereas influenza B and C viruses infect humans only, influenza A viruses also infect birds and other animals such as pigs. This unique ability to jump the species barrier enables influenza A viruses to cause pandemics.

Vaccines offer the best line of defense in reducing illness and deaths during a flu pandemic. However, currently available flu vaccines are likely to provide little or no immunity in a pandemic situation (although people who are due for their "ordinary" annual flu vaccine should still have one). A new vaccine must be developed to match the pandemic strain of virus. This work can only begin once that strain has been identified, although preparatory work can shorten the lead time in production.

This means that:

• Once a pandemic virus has been identified, even with the preparatory work under way, it will probably take around four to six months to produce a vaccine, possibly longer.

• Vaccines are unlikely to be available during the early stages of a pandemic and even then will not offer 100 percent protection.

• When a vaccine is available, the aim will be to immunize the whole population as quickly as possible as vaccine supplies increase.

• Manufacturers will not be able to produce enough vaccines to immunize everyone immediately. This means that vaccines will be given to some high-priority groups of people before others.

Medicines known as antivirals active against flu are the only other major medical countermeasure available. They may be used in the absence of, or as an adjunct to, vaccination. Antiviral drugs work by preventing the flu virus from reproducing. For treatment, they must be taken within forty-eight hours of the onset of symptoms in order to be effective. Antiviral drugs are expensive, take time to manufacture, have a limited shelf life, and will be in high international demand at the time of a pandemic. As with other medicines, it will be necessary to use them in the most effective way.

If a pandemic flu strain is causing outbreaks overseas, it will almost certainly reach the United States. Once it reaches our shores, it is expected to spread throughout the country in a matter of weeks, causing much more illness and higher death rates than those associated with "ordinary" flu. This will result in intense pressure on health care and other essential services and disruption to many aspects of daily life. It is currently impossible to predict when the flu pandemic will begin. It is also difficult to predict its impact with any accuracy.

Studies by the Centers for Disease Control and Prevention estimate between 2 million and 7.4 million deaths worldwide. The level of preparedness in each country will also influence the final death toll.

In high-income countries alone (including the United States), which represent 15 percent of the world's population, experts anticipate around 280,000 to 650,000 deaths, 134 million to 233 million hospital visits, and 1.55 million to 2 million hospital admissions. For planning purposes the World Health Organization advises that national pandemic plans be based on a cumulative clinical attack rate of 25 percent, compared to the attack rate of 5 percent to 10 percent associated with "ordinary" flu.

The National Strategy for Pandemic Influenza guides U.S. preparedness and response to an influenza pandemic, with the intent of (1) stopping, slowing or otherwise limiting the spread of a pandemic to the United States; (2) limiting the domestic spread of a pandemic, and mitigating disease, suffering and death; and (3) sustaining infrastructure and mitigating impact to the economy and the functioning of society.

The pillars of the Strategy are:

• Preparedness and Communication: Activities that should be undertaken before a pandemic to ensure preparedness, and the communication of roles and responsibilities to all levels of government, segments of society and individuals.

• Surveillance and Detection: Domestic and international systems that provide continuous "situational awareness," to ensure the earliest warning possible to protect the population.

• Response and Containment: Actions to limit the spread of the outbreak and to mitigate the health, social and economic impacts of a pandemic.

SEVERE ACUTE RESPIRATORY SYNDROME (SARS)

SARS is a viral respiratory illness caused by a coronavirus, called SARS-associated coronavirus (SARS-CoV). SARS was first reported in Asia in February 2003. The illness spread to more than two dozen countries in North America, South America, Europe, and Asia before the SARS global outbreak of 2003 was contained. Currently, there is no known SARS transmission anywhere in the world. The most recent human cases of

SARS-CoV infection were reported in China in April 2004 in an outbreak resulting from a laboratory-acquired infection.

According to the World Health Organization (WHO), a total of 8,098 people worldwide became sick with SARS during the 2003 outbreak. Of these, 774 died. In the United States, only eight people had laboratory evidence of SARS-CoV infection. All of these people had traveled to other parts of the world with SARS. The SARS outbreak is a reminder of just how quickly a contagious illness can go global.

The main way that SARS seems to spread is by close person-to-person contact. The virus that causes SARS is thought to be transmitted most readily by respiratory droplets (droplet spread) produced when an infected person coughs or sneezes. Droplet spread can happen when droplets from the cough or sneeze of an infected person are propelled a short distance (generally up to 3 feet) through the air and deposited on the mucous membranes of the mouth, nose, or eyes of persons who are nearby. The virus also can spread when a person touches a surface or object contaminated with infectious droplets and then touches his or her mouth, nose, or eye(s). In addition, it is possible that the SARS virus might spread more broadly through the air (airborne spread) or by other ways that are not now known.

In the context of SARS, close contact means having cared for or lived with someone with SARS or having direct contact with respiratory secretions or body fluids of a patient with SARS. Examples of close contact include kissing or hugging, sharing eating or drinking utensils, talking to someone within 3 feet, and touching someone directly. Close contact does not include activities like walking by a person or briefly sitting across a waiting room or office.

Symptoms

In general, SARS begins with a high fever (temperature greater than 100.4°F [>38.0°C]). Other symptoms may include headache, an overall feeling of discomfort, and body aches. Some people also have mild respiratory symptoms at the outset. About 10 percent to 20 percent of patients have diarrhea. After 2 to 7 days, SARS patients may develop a dry cough. Most patients develop pneumonia.

If transmission of SARS-CoV recurs, there are some common-sense precautions that you can take that apply to many infectious diseases. The most important is frequent hand washing with soap and water or use of an alcohol-based hand rub. You should also avoid touching your eyes, nose, and mouth with unclean hands and encourage people around you to cover their nose and mouth with a tissue when coughing or sneezing.

CDC continues to work with other federal agencies, state and local health departments, and healthcare organizations to plan for rapid recognition and response if person-to-person transmission of SARS-CoV recurs. CDC has developed recommendations and guidelines to help public health and healthcare officials plan for and respond quickly to the reappearance of SARS or other contagious illnesses and viruses.